The 30-Minute
Celebrity Makeover Miracle

Also by Steve Zim

6 Weeks to a Hollywood Body

Hot Point Fitness

The 30-Minute
Celebrity
Makeover
Miracle

Achieve the Body You've
Always Wanted

STEVE ZIM
with
STEVE STEINBERG

BICENTENNIAL
1807
WILEY
2007
BICENTENNIAL

John Wiley & Sons, Inc.

Published by John Wiley & Sons, Inc., Hoboken, New Jersey
Published simultaneously in Canada

All photographs by Nicolas Sage

Wiley Bicentennial Logo: Richard J. Pacifico

Design and composition by Navta Associates, Inc.

The information in this book is not intended to serve as a replacement for professional medical advice. Any use of the information in this book is at the reader's discretion. The author and the publisher specifically disclaim any and all liability arising directly or indirectly from the use or application of any information contained in this book. A health care professional should be consulted regarding your specfic situation.

For general information about our other products and services, please contact our Customer Care Department within the United States at (800) 762-2974, outside the United States at (317) 572-3993 or fax (317) 572-4002.

Wiley also publishes its books in a variety of electronic formats. Some content that appears in print may not be available in electronic books. For more information about Wiley products, visit our web site at www.wiley.com.

Library of Congress Cataloging-in-Publication Data:

Zim, Steve.
    The 30-minute celebrity makeover miracle : achieve the body you've always wanted / Steve Zim.
      p. cm.
    Includes index.
      ISBN 978-0-470-17403-6 (cloth : alk. paper)
    1. Exercise. 2. Physical fitness. 3. Bodybuilding. 4. Nutrition. 5. Celebrities—Health and hygiene. I. Title. II. Title: Thirty minute celebrity makeover miracle.
    RA781.Z538 2007
    613.7'1—dc22

                                                                                                  2007039343

Printed in the United States of America

10 9 8 7 6 5 4 3 2 1

To my mother, Cookie Zimelman, who is always in my heart.

Contents

Acknowledgments

Thanks to Tom Miller for shepherding this project from the beginning to the end. To Steve Steinberg, a great writer, who turned my words into a book. To Nicolas Sage for making my exercises pop off the page. To Maria Yip for her hard work producing great segments on the Weekend Today show and allowing me to educate millions of people about how to stay healthy. To Ivorie Anthony, Pat Robertson, and Kristi Watts at the 700 Club for allowing me to share my knowledge with their viewers. Thanks to the TV Guide Network for inviting me to explain how to really get a Hollywood Body. To Dennis Weiss for always making me think bigger. To Chuck Dalaklis, Teresa McKeown, Dennis and Sharon Dugan, and the Brokaw brothers—your support means the world to me. To Mel Berger, William Morris agent extraordinaire, for bringing Tom and me together. To Dr. Abraham Zimelman, my dad and medical adviser for my fitness segments, and Dr. Alice Zimelman. To Shirley Rubinstein for being more than family and always giving me great ideas for segments. To Irv Rubinstein for proving my theory correct by exercising and coming back from his stroke better and stronger than ever. To my wife, Jodi, who always supports me and is the best partner I could have ever dreamed of. To Carli and Taylor, who are the cutest gymnasts and sweetest daughters in the world. To Hank, my new running partner, for keeping me moving. To the gang at the gym: Salter Giddens, Chris Yackley, Alyson Sanders, Enrique Collazo, Danika DaMatta, and Deana Fletes. To the Wiley team: production editor Lisa

Burstiner and freelance copy editor Patti Waldygo. Last, but not least, to our models, Jodi Zimelman, Alyson Sanders, and Sarah Koplin.

Steve Zim

Thanks to Steve Zim for letting me be a part of his latest project, and thanks to these folks for keeping life fun while I was doing it: Anddy, Andre, Benny, Patrick, Michele, Sabunim, and Wendy.

Steve Steinberg

1

What Is the Celebrity Makeover Miracle?

Time—there's never enough of it. Most of us already have too much to do. We've gone beyond just burning the candle at both ends; our candles are fully engulfed in flames. Work, kids, school, shopping, cleaning. You get the picture. Sadly, when time gets tight, the first thing we sacrifice is taking proper care of ourselves. We try to get by on less sleep, we skip meals, and we cut back on the time we spend at the gym.

As a trainer, the two biggest questions I get are "Can I really change my body if I only have thirty minutes to work out?" and "Should I be doing cardio or lifting weights?" Happily, I know the answers to these questions. My job is to transform bodies. If there's one thing I know, it's makeovers. I've done them on the *Weekend Today* show, *Access Hollywood*, *Entertainment Tonight*, VH1, and the USA Network, to name just a few places. What makes these makeovers unlike the ones you see in magazines is that they are done on video, not in still pictures. Pictures can be studied and chosen to show off the model at his or her best. Unflattering shots end up in the trash, or they get touched up until they're more flattering. Video, on the other hand, doesn't lie. What you see is what you get.

When a TV crew comes into my gym, A Tighter U Fitness Studio, with cameras, they want to expose everything and see whether I can really pull off a seriously jaw-dropping makeover. My reputation is on the line every time, and thank God, I always get the job done.

Even though there's added pressure on me when I'm doing a makeover for a high-profile actor or actress, it's actually easier than doing a similar makeover on a regular person like you or me. They have more time and we don't. If I'm getting an actor ready for a part, he has six or eight weeks to get in shape. During that time, his only responsibilities are to learn a script and get in shape. He doesn't have to worry about wrapping up the year-end accounting numbers, waiting for the plumber to show up, or shuttling four kids to soccer practice, chess club, and karate class the way you do.

Doing these makeovers for people who aren't celebrities, as I do for many shows, is where I get some of my biggest thrills because most people don't think they can do it. These are normal people. They have jobs. They have kids. They don't have an entourage. And they don't have countless hours to work out every day. They may have 30 minutes a few days a week to exercise—and that's it. These makeovers get done—with dramatic results—because I understand that there are three vital components to a successful makeover: aerobics, strength training, and proper nutrition. All three are necessary to get your body to change quickly.

The strategies that I use in my TV makeovers are in this book, so you can get the same impressive results at home.

Cardio or Weight Lifting?

When most people work out, they either lift weights or do an aerobic activity like the treadmill or the elliptical. It's one or the other. But let's look at some numbers.

If you lift weights for 30 minutes, you can get your heart rate into the 50 to 55 percent range of its maximal rate. If you do cardio, you can raise your heart rate into the 65 to 80 percent range. What happens when we take the two activities and combine them? What if three days a week we did a cardio-weight program? These are rhetorical questions because I already know the answers: you lose weight, tone up, and look and feel great—all in just a half-hour only three days a week. I call it the 30-Minute Celebrity Makeover Miracle, and it's the ten-week program that I've used to transform celebrities and noncelebrities alike. How did this whole thing come about?

In the late eighties, I was a student at Boston College. My father had a doctor friend who was using cutting-edge infrared technology to track the progress of his patients recovering from injuries. My father knew I was into working out, and he figured that since the doctor's work involved muscles and working out involved muscles, a visit to this doctor's office would be the most exciting afternoon a twenty-year-old could possibly have.

After about an hour of watching the doctor scan patients to monitor blood flow into their various injured areas, I had an idea. I asked the doctor, "Is there any way this can be used to track blood flow during exercise?" I told him that a lot of the time when I worked out, I didn't feel things where I knew I was supposed to—my muscles didn't feel the way I thought they should. Was it because I wasn't doing the exercises correctly? Or maybe the exercises weren't as good as they could be.

We used very expensive equipment to test a standard overhead shoulder press—the press that everyone considers the ultimate shoulder exercise. What we came up with was interesting. The blood didn't flow into the shoulder as much as I'd expected. It flowed to the tops of the shoulders, the triceps (along the backs of the arms), and the lats (the large muscles of the back).

I played around a bit and came up with an exercise called W Shoulders (which you'll be doing soon), and bang! When we looked at the movements under the infrared scan, we found that all the blood ran into the shoulder. I was hooked. I came up with a list of other exercises that performed just as well under the scan. I added them to my workout and saw my body begin to change. People started asking me about the exercises I was doing. When I told them, they did these exercises and began to see results, too. That was the beginning of my teaching this program.

Around the same time, I made some interesting observations about the cardio I saw people do at the gym. There was the guy who went all out. You know the type—he goes crazy for about ten minutes and then stops because he can't maintain it. He'd be at the gym for about two weeks, and then I wouldn't see him again for months. Eventually, I'd run into him, and he'd give me a handful of excuses but say that he'd be back at the gym real soon. A few months later, he'd show up at the gym, and the same thing would happen again.

And then there was a woman I called the mall-walker. She burned up the treadmill at a scorching half-mile-an-hour pace. You know those special effects in *The Matrix* when they moved in super–slow motion to dodge bullets? The mall-walkers were slower, much slower. Sure, they were on the treadmills every day, but their bodies never seemed to change. They read a ton of magazines while they walked, which made them smarter, but that was about it. If you're going so slow that you can read, then you're not working hard enough. The mall-walkers don't put in the effort they need to make their bodies change.

There were also the folks who ran at a steady pace that challenged them but didn't kill them. They weren't there every day, but that's because they didn't have to be. Their bodies were changing, and they were able to make that happen in a safe and doable way. It made me think of the fairy tale about the tortoise and the hare, and I realized that in real life neither of them would have won the race. If there had been a third animal in the race—one that ran not too slow and not too fast—it would have been the winner.

Fast forward a few years. Now I'm in my gym in Los Angeles using these theories and exercises on my clients and getting astounding results. I have had athletes who weren't even Olympic hopefuls make it to the Olympics, minor league baseball players who wound up playing in major league stadiums, and actors and actresses who hadn't been able to change their bodies suddenly slimming down, becoming leaner, and landing roles. And I've worked with plenty of new moms who thought that after having babies they would have to live with their new shapes. Not only did I get them back into their old clothes and into the physical condition that enabled them to keep up with their kids, most of them actually looked better than they had before they were pregnant!

So how does it work?

Cardio and Weight Lifting

By combining your aerobic and strength training and making sure that every activity you do is getting the absolute most out of your body, you're keeping your heart rate up so that you don't have to do any extra cardio. You're also doing weight-bearing exercises to strengthen your body and help to build lean muscle. You'll burn more calories while you work out by keeping your heart rate up, and, even more important, thanks to the strength training, you'll increase the rate at which your body burns calories over the next 24 to 48 hours as it works to rebuild healthier and stronger muscle fibers.

Let's break it down some more. Say your body likes to burn 1,800 calories a day. This is without exercise or any other heavy physical activity. It's just the calories your body burns doing the everyday things it does, such as keeping your heart beating and your lungs pumping, walking up the stairs, petting the dog, and so on. If you eat 1,800 calories and you burn 1,800 calories, you won't gain any weight and you won't lose weight. Over time, though, if you don't exercise, your lean muscle mass—the amount of lean muscle on your body— will start to deteriorate. As it diminishes, so does your ability to burn calories. You'll burn fewer and fewer calories every day. Soon, your body will burn only 1,700 calories a day. If you eat 1,800 calories a day, you're packing away 100 extra calories a day. If you eat 100 calories a day more than your body needs for an entire year, you will gain 10½ pounds of fat. That's the bad news.

The good news is that if you exercise with weights and build your lean muscle mass, you can flip that equation upside-down. Every additional pound of lean muscle you build forces your body to burn between 35 and 50 calories more per day than it would otherwise. If, over the course of a year, you gain 10 pounds of lean muscle mass—not bulk, but lean muscle—your body will burn 350 to 500 more calories per day than it would have. If your body now burns 2,200 calories a day, and you're eating that same 1,800 calories, it will tap into the stored energy (aka fat) that you have on your body for the other 400 calories, and you'll start to lose weight quickly.

Want even more good news? With the 30-Minute Celebrity Makeover Miracle, you'll push your heart rate up near 80 percent of its maximum. Since the higher your heart rate, the more calories you burn, this will let you burn the greatest amount of calories in the least amount of time. And you'll be doing it safely.

Keeping your heart rate at that 80 percent rate by doing cardio alone can be pretty intense, and, over time, you will have a greater chance of being injured. With my program, you're multitasking, and while your heart rate may be right up at 80 percent, it doesn't feel like it. It's much easier to keep your heart rate up by combining strength training and cardio than it is by doing weight training or aerobic work alone. As a result, your body feels like it's working less, your heart doesn't know the difference—all it knows is that it's working at 80 percent—and you're burning calories like nobody's business. Add these calories you burn during the workout to the increased number that your body now burns every day as a result of your strength training, and you move that much closer and faster to a new you—again, all in only a half-hour three days a week. (Of course, if you want to add some other cardio on the days you're not doing my workout, feel free. Swimming, hiking, and fast walking are all great ways to bump up the number of calories you burn during the week.)

Nutrition

That brings us to the third piece of the puzzle. If you're lifting weights and doing your cardio but not eating well, yes, you'll get results, but not nearly as quickly and not with that wow factor you're shooting for. To lose weight and make sure that it's fat, not muscle, that you're losing, you have to eat correctly. Weight loss, at its core, is about a simple equation: intake versus expenditure. There needs to be a deficit between the calories that you take in and those you burn off.

My program goes beyond making sure that you eat the right number of calories. I'll show you that all calories were not created equally and how, by using the glycemic index, you can optimize the fat-burning capabilities of your own body. I'll teach you the tricks I use when doing makeovers to guarantee that you lose weight without starving yourself. You'll be surprised at just how much—and how often—you'll be eating. And you won't have to give up your favorite foods. You'll lose body fat safely and without feeling deprived.

A New You in 10 Weeks

What can you expect when you put together all three pieces of the puzzle—strength training, cardiovascular conditioning, and proper nutrition?

The answer is up to you. I live in Southern California, and a lot of my clients—even those who aren't actors and actresses—have developed a Hollywood mentality. They want to make the most of themselves. Everyone wants to be a star. This could mean being the star of a $200 million blockbuster movie or simply being the star of his or her own life. No actor ever strutted into Hollywood with the ultimate goal of someday landing the lead role in a dishwashing detergent ad. Stars want to make it big, really big, with their names listed above the titles of their movies. The best and most dedicated of them achieve that goal.

I'm giving you a fitness blueprint for an incredibly efficient way of making the most out of yourself, but, ultimately, it's up to you. If you're willing to put in the time and effort for the next ten weeks, you will be rewarded. Within one week, you'll notice differences in your body, and within two weeks, your friends and coworkers will start asking what you've been doing to look so good. I'll be honest and tell you up front that there will be days when you won't feel like working out or moments when you might even want to quit. Even half an hour can seem like an eternity sometimes. But that's when you'll have to dig deep and find the strength to keep going. What you put into it is what you'll get out of it.

My program has worked for thousands of clients, and I know it can work for you. So let's turn the page and get started.

2

Celebrity Makeover Strength

Look at Jessica Alba, Jessica Simpson, or Jennifer Garner. Or, as proof that all hope isn't lost after forty, look at Madonna. They have the Hollywood body. These women aren't just thin and sexy; they're lean, muscular, and sexy. They're strong. That doesn't happen by mistake. These women know that the road to the celebrity look goes straight through the weight room.

For men, lifting weights has always been part of getting in shape and looking their best, but for women, that hasn't always been the case. The curvy, more voluptuous shape that was popular in the forties and fifties gave way to the twig-thin figure that fashion models sported in the sixties and seventies. Did these women strength train? No. But if you ignore these trendy and dated looks and focus on pure beauty, you learn some pretty interesting things.

Women and Weights

When women tell me they're scared to lift weights because it will bulk them up and make them look like NFL linebackers, I bring them into my office and show them one of my favorite pictures. It's a shot of Marilyn Monroe lying on a bench doing dumbbell chest presses. You can see the definition around her shoulders, triceps, and pecs and the sexy way her upper body tapers down to a slim waist. Yes, Marilyn Monroe—one of the most beautiful women ever—lifted.

Muscle is your best weapon when it comes to burning fat. The fat on your body doesn't do a whole lot. It's like your kids when they're on school vacation, just sitting around doing nothing. Muscle, on the other hand, is living, breathing tissue. It needs nutrients to survive. For every pound of sexy lean muscle that you add to your body, you will burn an extra 35 to 50 calories per day.

But muscle does more than merely increase your day-to-day calorie burn. Contrary to what you may think, when you lift weights, you don't build your muscles; you tear them down. It's over the next 24 to 48 hours that the actual building takes place. Your body has to fix the damage you did and make your muscles stronger so that they will be better able to handle your workouts. All that rebuilding burns even more calories. All of my workouts are full-body workouts. They're designed to work as many of your body's muscles as possible to take full advantage of this residual calorie burn. Weight training will turn your body into a calorie-burning—and fat-burning—machine. Marilyn knew what she was doing!

For women, the strength training that we will do won't turn you into a behemoth. There are a couple of reasons for this. First, we will be doing a fitness weight routine and not a bodybuilding weight routine. You'll lift lighter weights and do more repetitions. If I was preparing you for a pro wrestling career, which I'm not, you would be lifting far heavier weights and doing fewer reps.

Second, women are not men. Chemically, your bodies are not designed to develop large muscles. Men have much more testosterone flowing through their bodies than you do. As a result, you won't develop the body and the musculature of a man. And here are a couple of other things that men do but you won't because of your lower testosterone levels: you won't get insanely mad because the cable isn't working, you won't throw your 6-iron into the woods because you sliced your fairway shot, and you won't get into an argument with someone who gets in the "eight items or fewer" line at the supermarket with nine items. In summary, my weight-lifting program will not turn you into a hulk. Be thankful you're not a man.

Men and Women Need to Fight Osteoporosis

If you're a man, even though you might think you don't have to read the next three paragraphs, you really do.

Osteoporosis happens when your bones get weak and brittle. Most people think it's a disease that only women get. Twenty percent of those suffering from osteoporosis are men. One of the best ways to stave off the disease or reduce its impact is by doing weight-bearing exercise. Walking and jogging are both great weight-bearing exercises. Your body has to support itself (bear its own weight) while you move. Strength training, though, is tops when it comes to weight-bearing exercises. Numerous studies have shown that weight lifting can reverse the effects of osteoporosis by increasing bone density.

The explanation for this phenomenon is that your bones are in a constant state of regeneration. As old bone cells die, new ones appear. In fact, your whole skeleton regenerates itself over a 10-year period. Bone cells, though, regenerate only at the strength they need to, in order to do what you ask of them. The less you ask them to do, the weaker they grow back. Over time, your bones get weaker and weaker. You start to walk all hunched over. A slight fall, which 10 years earlier you would have easily brushed off, can shatter a leg, an arm, or a hip bone. While you recover, you're asking even less of your bone cells so they continue to get weaker and weaker. It's a very bad and dangerous cycle to be in.

Suppose, though, you begin to lift weights. Now, all of a sudden, you're asking a lot of your bones. You're asking them to support not only your own weight, but the additional weight of dumbbells. When your bone cells start to regenerate, they need to be stronger, not weaker, than their predecessors. As you get stronger, thanks to your strength training, you will be lifting heavier weights and thus requiring your bone cells to grow back even stronger. This is the cycle that you want to be in. Weight training can actually help to reverse the aging process when it comes to your bones.

Men and Weights

For men, the Hollywood body began with the actor Johnny Weissmuller when he played Tarzan. He was big, strong, and muscular, and in 1932 every man wanted to look like that. Heck, why not? There was Weissmuller, swinging around the jungle with a scantily clad Maureen O'Sullivan on his arm. Not a bad Depression-era fantasy.

The celebrity look has always been about fantasy. Muscularity represented sexuality. The good-looking, strong, and muscular guys always got the girl. Think of Burt Lancaster in *From Here to Eternity* or Marlon Brando in any of his early roles. The thing about the Hollywood body of the thirties, the forties, and the early fifties was that it was an achievable look. If you ate right and did your push-ups and pull-ups, you could look like that.

In the late fifties, things started to change. A bodybuilder named Steve Reeves hit the screen as Hercules. Women swooned, and men realized they would have to do more than simple calisthenics to keep up. The fantasy was becoming more and more of just that: a fantasy.

The fantasy of having the Hollywood body seemed dashed for good in 1970, when a young Austrian bodybuilder made his screen debut in, ironically, another Hercules movie, *Hercules in New York*. Arnold Schwarzenegger, already a multiple Mr. Universe winner, was unlike anyone the screen had ever seen before. For the next thirty years, that look—giant pecs, massive arms, and so on—was the Hollywood body. Fueled by visions of looking like Arnold or like Sylvester Stallone when he got all buff in *Rocky III*, guys hit the gym. And they hit it hard.

What happened? Everyone wanted to be huge, but no one really knew how. Men would work on only the muscles they could see in the mirror: all chest and arm exercises and no back or leg work. Sure, they ended up with decent-sized pecs, biceps, and triceps, but because of the unbalanced way they worked their bodies, they were a complete mess otherwise. Their shoulders curled in and they walked all hunched over, with spindly legs doing their best to support oddly oversized upper bodies. A real sexy image, huh? Hasta la vista, baby!

But for the moviegoer, it wasn't long before big wasn't big enough. In 2003, director Ang Lee brought Marvel Comics' Incredible Hulk to the silver screen for the first time. Did Lee use Arnold in the lead role? Did he call up Lou Ferrigno, who played the green giant on TV? Did he phone bodybuilder Ronnie Coleman, who might just be the biggest and most muscular man on the planet? No. He decided to use an entirely computer-generated Hulk. The movie strongman, the icon who had been the Hollywood body for the last thirty years, was no longer the result of pumping iron; it was the result of crunching numbers.

Today's Hollywood Body

Happily, the Hollywood body has come full circle. Today's Hollywood body for men and women is muscular but lean. It stresses tone over bulk, a six-pack over big pecs and biceps. It's Brad Pitt. It's Matt Damon in *The Bourne Identity* and its sequels. It's Daniel Craig as James Bond. And, for maybe the first time in a couple of generations, it's an achievable look. Yes, we're trying to look like humans again.

Lifting weights will improve your metabolism so you'll burn more calories throughout the day. If you're a woman, it will give you sexy-looking tone and definition. If you're a man, it will add some size to that tone and definition. It will help you to avoid osteoporosis or will lessen the effects of the disease if you already have it.

Now, it's time to lift the darn things.

Strength Training—the Right Way

Like everything else about my 30-Minute Celebrity Makeover Miracle, the strength training you do will be simple, straightforward, and effective. We will focus on three things: making sure that you do the right exercises, making sure that you use the right form, and making sure that you use the right weights.

How do you choose the right exercises? That's easy. Follow my workout-by-workout guide for the entire 10-week program.

The body needs to be worked in a balanced way. If you work the left side, you need to work the right side. If you work the front, you have to work the back. If you work the top, you have to work the bottom. If you do a pushing motion—like a chest press—you have to balance it with a pulling motion, like a row. If you do a flexing motion, like a biceps curl, you have to balance it with an extending motion, like a triceps kickback, for example. My program is balanced, so you are balanced.

The exercises you'll do were designed to keep you in balance and reduce any imbalances that your body may already have. But aside from the aesthetic advantage of working out in a balanced fashion, such as looking more proportional and having fewer obvious "weak" spots, there are some very practical reasons for working out like this. By making sure that you offset your pushing motions with pulling motions and by working the shoulders correctly, you'll improve your posture. Simply improving your posture will make you stand taller. In addition to making you taller, and thereby appear thinner, an improved posture will deepen your breathing and will lessen your chances of developing back pain.

You'll also decrease the strength differences between your weak and strong sides. If you're right-handed, I bet there are things you can do only with your right hand. That's a limitation we're going to remove. Working with dumbbells, as you'll be doing, is a great way to achieve this. If you have to do a single-arm biceps curl with a dumbbell, there's nothing your right arm can do to help your left arm. Your left side is forced to get stronger. You want to be able to do anything with your weak side that you can do with your strong side, and I'll help you to do just that.

The exercises also make the most of your time by letting you stretch your body as you strengthen it. Your body is designed with muscles that oppose each other. It's how the body stabilizes itself. Your chest muscles in the front of your body oppose your back muscles. This is how the shoulders are stabilized. Conveniently, when you do a pushing motion, like a chest press or a push-up, to strengthen the chest, you actually stretch the muscles in the back at the same time. Try it for yourself right where you are. Using both arms, imagine that you're pushing open a very heavy door. In addition to feeling your chest muscles contract, you can probably also feel a stretch taking place across your back. Everything you'll do in my program is designed to stretch as it strengthens.

But the most important thing is that these have to be exercises you can actually do. Here's one of the biggest mistakes people make in the gym. They see an article in a magazine that tells them to stand on a stability ball and do one-handed shoulder presses with their eyes closed. Sure, the article was written for elite, world-class circus performers, but people figure that since they've been going to the gym for almost a month, they can handle it, but the truth is, they can't.

The exercises you'll do in my program gradually ramp up in difficulty. As you progress through the weeks, you'll be given more challenging things to do. I start you off simply because you have to walk before you can run. (And you will literally be walking before you run, but more about that in the cardio chapter.) Don't be lulled into a false sense of security, however, if some of the initial exercises seem easy. I'm no pushover. You will be challenged. And don't worry if there's an exercise that you can't do or have trouble with. The exercise section of my book is divided by body part, so simply substitute another exercise that works the same body part for the exercise you have trouble with. Can't seem to do the Hollywood Arrows? No problem. Just substitute some Hollywood Butt Kicks in their place.

The ever-increasing number of exercises that you'll learn also serves another purpose: they'll keep your body, and you, from getting bored. If you've ever joined a gym and been given an initial consultation where someone hands you a list of eight or ten exercises to do, you know what I mean. You stick with the routine for a couple of weeks, and you might even see some changes happening to your body, but then what happens? Your body stops changing, and you get discouraged. In addition to that, you're bored with doing the same things over and over again. So what happens? You stop exercising.

Achieving fitness means that your body must adapt to new movements and situations. If you stick with the same handful of exercises, your body will stop responding. By constantly hitting you with new exercises and having you do some of the older exercises in different orders, I keep your body constantly on its toes, in a state of shock and surprise. You never hit plateaus where your body stops changing, and you never get bored with doing the same workout again and again.

The Right Form

How do you know you're doing the exercises with the right form? In an ideal world, I'd be standing beside you to show you how to do each exercise, but here you're getting the next-best thing. I've given you a full-page description of every exercise, along with pictures, a discussion of the correct technique, and tips about things to look for and things to avoid. I've described them here the way I describe them to my clients.

A few things that pictures can't convey, though, concern breathing, stability, and control. You should understand all of them to get the most out of your workout.

It's not enough to simply breathe. Yes, you'll stay alive, but you won't be taking advantage of the power of inhaling and exhaling at the proper times. In every exercise, there's a positive phase and a negative phase. For example, take the Hollywood Hammer Curls for your biceps. When you raise the weight up from waist height to shoulder height, that's the positive phase. That's when you're exerting yourself the most. It's important that you always breathe out—exhale—on exertion. When you lower the weight back to the starting position, that's the negative phase, and that's when you need to inhale. It may sound simple, but you'd be amazed by the difference it makes in your performance when you breathe correctly. I've had clients who normally could do only 10 repetitions of chest presses with a certain weight, and all of a sudden they crank out 12 or 15 reps with that same weight by doing nothing more than closely monitoring their breathing.

I'm even going to tell you how to breathe. Most people breathe into their chests. That's fine. It does the job of getting oxygen into your system. You could live very happily just breathing into your chest. But have you ever seen how a baby or a small child breathes? You can see the air going all the way down into his belly. His stomachs inflates like a mini-balloon. That's the way I want you to breathe before every set of exercises. Take one of those deep breaths that you feel all the way down to your lower abdomen, hold it, and then pull your belly button in as if you were trying to touch it to your spine. After that, I just want you to breathe normally while you keep visualizing your belly button being pulled toward your spine.

What you've done is to connect your upper body with your lower body. You've loaded your diaphragm and created a cylinder of power that will keep you solid from your shoulders all the way down to your ankles. This cylinder is reinforced strength that will allow you to get the most out of each exercise and protect your spine and your lower back from potential injury.

I recently had a sixty-year-old man come to see me. He wasn't a regular client of mine, but he knew about the kinds of things I did with my clients and the results they can achieve. He had been active and healthy all his life, until about a month earlier. He had noticed he was losing strength. He went to see his doctor and was diagnosed with a very bad case of rheumatoid arthritis. Soon, every motion became difficult and painful. He had gone from being strong and self-sufficient to being very close to an invalid in really just the blink of an eye. He sat on a chair in front of me and I had him do the very same breathing technique I just explained. He took a deep breath into his stomach, pulled his belly button in and, for the first time in a month, was able to get up out of the chair by himself and without any pain. Individually, his muscles weren't strong enough to get him out of the chair, but by connecting everything, he was able to harness the strength to stand up by himself. His body was working in concert with itself. He was so thrilled he gave me the biggest hug and the wettest kiss I think I've ever received.

You're also going to use this concept of connecting the various parts of your body to keep your neck safe and help you maximize the results from your core and abdominal work, or just about any exercise that you do lying on your back. And it's incredibly simple. I want you to try something. Place the palm of your right hand against the back of your head and gently push it forward. What happened? Your head lolled forward like you were a bobble-head doll, right? Now I want you to take the tip of your tongue and place it against the inside of your upper front teeth. Try pushing your head forward again. Now, instead of your head just coming forward, your entire upper body did. Just as you did with the breathing technique, you've created a cylinder of strength that has connected your head with your upper body. If you've always shied away from abdominal exercises because you've felt them more in your neck than in your midsection, your worries are over. By concentrating on small things like breathing and tongue placement, you're able to add strength and stability to your entire body. Now we just have to make sure you have good control.

If you've ever seen the guy at the gym—and it's always a guy— who swings the weights around as he lifts, his body pitching forward and bending backward as he strains to keep from falling over, you've seen someone who's out of control. He thinks he's getting a great workout—"Look at the heavy weights I'm using!"—but he's really not. He's not targeting the muscles he thinks he is, and he's a prime candidate for getting injured. It's not about how much you lift; it's how well you lift. Let's go back to the biceps curl. To take full advantage of the positive phase of the exercise, when you're lifting the weight to your shoulder (and exhaling), you want to make sure that your biceps are doing the work. This means you can't throw your hips forward, lean back, bounce your knees, and so on. You need to control and stabilize your body and force your biceps to do all of the work.

Just as important is the negative phase. Sure, it's easy to just let the weight fall back into the starting position by letting your arm go slack, but if you do, you're missing out on half the benefits of the exercise. By lowering the weight slowly back to the starting position, you're continuing to work your biceps. I have my clients lift the weight to a one-beat count and lower it to a two-beat count. They have to come to a dead stop at the starting position before they do another rep, to make sure they're using their muscles, and not just momentum, to do the work. It's my "Bring it, don't swing it" approach to lifting.

The Right Weight

How do you know you're using the right weight? Once again, that's easy. When it comes to the way you'll be lifting weights, the 30-Minute Celebrity Makeover Miracle differs from just about any other strength-training program you've ever tried. Most weight routines will have you doing two to three sets of somewhere between 10 and 15 repetitions of an exercise. You'll do, for example, a set of 12 squats, rest for a bit, do another set of 12, rest, and then do the final set. My program is about strength training, but it also focuses on keeping your heart rate up. You'll do only one set of any exercise per workout, but it will based on time, rather than on a given number of repetitions. Every set is a minute long.

You'll be lifting lighter weights than you may be used to, because a minute is a long time. You'll want to choose a weight (and it will be different for just about every exercise) that you can do at a consistent pace for the entire minute. The key is that I want the last 10 seconds of each minute to be a challenge. If you just blow through the repetitions as if you were holding a pencil, the weight is too light and your body won't respond because it's not being challenged. If the weight is too heavy, you won't be able to lift for a minute straight with perfect form. Your heart rate will drop lower than we want, and you'll also increase your risk of getting injured from doing the motions incorrectly.

What's great about the formula is that it works perfectly for both men and women. Men will use a proportionally heavier weight than women will, but it's still a weight that they can lift for an entire minute. Lifting a heavier weight will let them add size to their muscles while still keeping their heart rate up and their bodies burning fat. Women will lift a much lighter weight for that lean and muscular look.

Here's a tip I give my clients when they're not sure about what weight to use. Once you've chosen your weight, make sure you have a pair of slightly heavier dumbbells and a pair of slightly lighter dumbbells within easy reach. If you're doing, say, the Hollywood Overhead Tris and after the first 15 seconds you think it's too easy, quickly grab the heavier set. On the other hand, if you get to the 45-second mark and your arms are about to fall off, grab the lighter set and finish with those. And what if even your lightest dumbbells become too heavy toward the end of the minute? Simply put them down and finish off the minute doing the motion without any weights in your hands. I want you to keep moving and keep challenging yourself, even if this means working out without any dumbbells.

Don't get discouraged, though, if you have to drop to a lighter weight or use no weight at all. Ironically, this isn't a sign of weakness; it's a sign of strength. It shows that your muscles are working so hard that they are becoming fatigued. This is what you want. With clients I see on an ongoing basis (as opposed to the ones I have doing a turbo-charged program like the 30-Minute Celebrity Makeover Miracle), all of the work we do in the weight room is done "to failure." This means that they'll do a set of exercises until they can't do another repetition with perfect form. I'll admit it can be a tough sell to try to motivate someone when the ultimate goal is failure, but as long as my clients understand that failure is referring to their muscles under stress and not to them as people, it makes sense. If you've worked so hard that your muscles can't do another repetition, that's how you know that you're challenging them and that you're progressing.

Even better, and what really makes this program so effective, is that here you don't just stop and go out for coffee when you've reached that point. You grab a lighter weight and keep doing repetitions. When that weight becomes too heavy, you continue without any dumbbells at all. The result is that you've gone to failure multiple times in the same set. It's an incredible way to build strength and lean muscle.

Hey, I'm a Little Sore

Early on, especially if you've never attempted a training program before, you may feel some soreness a day or two after you work out. This is completely normal. It's your body's way of telling you that it's moving in new ways and is responding to the program. Remember, when you lift weights, you're actually tearing down the muscle. These microtears are the soreness that you're feeling. Feel free to take a couple of ibuprofens or apply some topical pain-relief cream if you want. Because you are sticking with lighter weights and doing more repetitions, you will greatly avoid the risk of injury that's often caused by trying to lift too much weight. A sharp pain that you feel while you're working out is not good and is more likely to occur during a bodybuilding workout than during the type of fitness workout that you're doing, but this delayed onset muscle soreness is something you may experience.

An interesting note about next-day soreness: women, especially, often misinterpret this soreness. They tell me after their first day of doing squats that their pants feel tighter. They believe this is a sure sign that their thighs are growing at an exponential rate and that they should cease all strength training before they are too large to be able to fit through my doorway. I explain to them that their legs did not grow from a single day of squats; if that's the way human bodies worked, each of my legs would have its own zip code. What happened was that the soreness from doing this new movement made their legs more sensitive to the touch. The women were actually more aware of the way their pants felt against their legs. The pants weren't any tighter; their legs were just more sensitive.

The strength training you do by lifting weights lays the foundation for the program. It builds the muscle that'll give you the strong but lean look that you want. The more lean muscle you add to your body—again, it won't be bulky muscle—the more calories your body will burn 24 hours a day. The next step is to keep things going by burning large numbers of calories in the shortest amount of time. And that's where your cardio comes in.

3

Celebrity Makeover Cardio

If, historically, strength training has been the domain of men, cardiovascular training has been the domain of women. That still holds true to some degree. Check out the cardio classes at your local gym, and you'll see mostly women in there. How did this come about?

In 1982, Jane Fonda came out with her first workout tape. It was designed to get you up, moving, and burning calories—and it was aimed at women. Men might have watched the video of pretty women jumping around, but they weren't playing along at home. While women burned their calories in leg warmers and headbands, men were happier lifting weights incorrectly in the weight room.

In the mid-eighties, that started to change. In the 1985 movie *Perfect*, John Travolta played a reporter who ends up investigating the seamy underbelly of the red-hot Los Angeles fitness scene. The movie was to the aerobics world what *Saturday Night Fever* had been to the disco world eight years earlier. The message, which was not lost on men, was that aerobics were on fire and that not only would you end up with the perfect body, but it would greatly increase your odds of meeting women with perfect bodies.

Here's the problem. An issue of *Rolling Stone* came out around the same time the movie did. On the cover was Travolta and costar Jamie Lee Curtis. Even though Curtis gave away a few inches to the taller Travolta, she looked like she outweighed him by around 15 pounds, and she carried barely an ounce of body fat! What were we thinking? Travolta had the "perfect" body? In the picture, it looked like his cheekbones were going to poke through the skin on his face. Someone get this guy some food!

In 1985, Travolta was the anti-Arnold. Where Arnold and his cantaloupelike pecs represented one end of the extreme fitness spectrum, the frail Travolta represented the other. People were doing their cardio, but they were doing too much of it. As a result, they weren't just burning fat; they were burning muscle. And they weren't looking all that healthy.

In 1968, Dr. Kenneth Cooper wrote his groundbreaking book *Aerobics*. Cooper coined the word *aerobics*. In his book, Cooper stressed the importance of exercises like walking, running, biking, and swimming. His case was that anything that improved your overall cardiovascular system—your heart and your lungs—would lead to a greater quality of life and a longer life expectancy. Did he, in his wildest dreams, imagine that this belief would someday lead to a magazine cover showing a scrawny Travolta? Probably not.

The Benefits of Cardio

The 30-Minute Celebrity Makeover Miracle uses cardio for two main reasons: to strengthen your cardiovascular system and to burn a lot of calories in a short time. You will not be doing marathon sessions of cardio. You'll use it wisely, in moderation.

Just as the skeletal muscles of your body—your lats, quads, biceps, and so on—get stronger when you continuously challenge them, the muscles of your heart also get stronger from a continuous challenge. What will a stronger heart do for you? Here are a few scientific facts.

Your heart started beating before you were born, and it will beat right up until the time you leave this world. Let's say it beats 70 times per minute. Multiply that by 60 and you get 4,200 beats per hour. In a day, that's more than 100,000 beats. In a year, it's close to 37 million beats. You want to live until you're ninety? Your heart will have to beat almost 3.5 billion times. And that figure of 70 beats per minute was your heart rate at rest. Walking, running, getting angry, or getting scared all raise your heart rate significantly. Just to be on the safe side, you have to make sure your heart is ready to handle 4 billion beats if you want to see age ninety.

Every beat of your heart pumps blood back into your system. The blood carries oxygen and important nutrients to your muscles, organs, and other body parts. By strengthening your heart, you'll be able to pump more blood into your system with each beat. Since the amount of blood your body needs doesn't change much, the more blood you can pump with each beat, the fewer times you'll have to pump. Your body will still get everything it needs, but your heart won't have to work as hard because it is stronger. Over time, cardio-vascular exercise will lower your resting heart rate by making your heart more efficient.

Let's look at the numbers again. If you can get your resting heart rate down to 60 (and with hard work, you can get it even lower), that brings your heartbeats per day down to around 86,000. That's 14,000 fewer beats per day, every day. Over a year, that's a reduction of more than 5 million beats. By getting your heart in shape, you can signifi- cantly reduce the amount of work it has to do to keep you alive. If you're planning to live to a ripe old age, you want to get your resting heart rate as low as you can.

A good way to test how strong your heart is getting as you go through the program is by monitoring your resting heart rate. Find a time of the day when you are relaxed and have been sitting for a while. Take your index and middle fingers and place them on the palm side of your opposite wrist, about two inches down from the base of the hand. Feel around until you feel something pulsing. That's your radial artery. Without pressing too hard, count how many times it pulses in a minute. Think about sitting on the beach, in a boat on a lake, or whatever else you find calming. Do this three times, then average your results. For example, if the first minute was 66, the second was 72, and the third was 70, that would average 69.3. We would round that down to 69. This would be your resting heart rate. The average person's resting heart rate is somewhere between 60 and 80. Use the worksheet in chapter 5 to fill in your initial resting heart rate. I've included worksheets at the end of each two-week phase of the 30-Minute Celebrity Makeover Miracle to let you easily monitor how strong your heart gets over the course of 10 weeks.

The Five Phases of Celebrity Makeover Cardio

Just as with the strength exercises, it's important to continually challenge and surprise your body. With your weight training, you did it by adding in new exercises over time, shuffling the order in which you worked your muscles, and increasing the weight you lifted as your body adapted and got stronger. For your cardio, you'll do the same thing.

You're going to ramp things up over the next 10 weeks, and it will start very simply: with walking. Walking may sound easy—you've been doing it since before you can remember. But if you haven't been involved in a fitness program for a while, alternating your strength training with 2 minutes of walking may be tough. Even if you have been working out, mixing in weight training with your cardio will make walking for 2 minutes seem harder than you think. If at any point, though, you're having trouble keeping up, slow it down or take a break. Different people will advance at different rates, so don't get discouraged if you think you can't keep up. You may be able to walk for only 30 seconds of the 2 minutes. That's fine. Eventually that 30 seconds becomes a full minute, and eventually 1 minute becomes 2 minutes. Just do your best.

At some point, the walking workout will become easy. I want it to. This shows that your cardiovascular system is getting stronger, that it's made adaptations to the challenges you're throwing at it. It's time to move on. Then we go to marching. You'll alternate minutes of weight lifting with minutes of marching in place. When that becomes routine, it's on to jogging, and then to stepping up on a stair or a platform, and then finally to lunging. It's a gradual progression that takes you from a very basic movement like walking and evolves into a very challenging move like lunging. The stronger your cardiovascular system gets, the harder we can push it. The harder we push it, the more calories you burn. That's why my program is so effective.

But the key is to do things gradually. If I started you off with the lunging phase of the program, you'd try it a couple of times, get discouraged, and then slowly limp over to my gym in Southern California and bounce this book off my forehead. But because we're increasing the intensity slowly over a 10-week period, you'll be able to handle the lunging phase when you get to it.

The fun part comes at the end of the 10 weeks. Not only will you look and feel great, but if you go back and do one of the first walking workouts in the program, one that was probably a challenge when you first tried it, you'll be amazed at how easy it is.

Some people, due to an injury or a chronic condition, may not be able to do one or more of the different phases. Don't worry, it's not the end of the world. In fact, it's far from it. I worked with an actress who was recovering from a serious knee injury but still needed to get into dynamite shape for a role. She couldn't jog in place or do lunges, so we worked around her condition by doing only walking, marching, and stepping for her cardio. She did the strength exercises from all five phases but let her body dictate which of the cardio exercises she did. After 10 weeks she looked fabulous.

Do what you can do and listen to your body. Even if you can only walk in place, if you work hard and are consistent, you'll see results. The key is to keep at it and always be positive. You may even end up surprising yourself. Your body may not be ready to move to the marching phase at the beginning of week 3, but by not giving up and by continuing to strengthen your body with walking, you may be ready for marching sooner than you thought.

Your Perfect Heart Rate

One problem that people have when they do cardio is not keeping their heart rates in the optimal range. My program guarantees that you'll work at the perfect intensity level. Remember the mall-walkers and how their bodies never seemed to change, even though they were on the treadmill every single day? Their bodies weren't changing because they weren't working hard enough. To really tap into your body's excess fat, you need to have your heart rate in the 60 to 80 percent range of your maximal heart rate.

While you could spend a small fortune going through a battery of tests to discover your body's maximal heart rate, we'll use a formula that's been shown to be pretty reliable. Take your age and subtract it from 220. If you're forty, that means your maximal heart rate is 180. If you're 60, it's 160.

To find the 60 to 80 percent range, take your maximal heart rate and multiply it by 0.6. Then take your maximal heart rate and multiply it by 0.8. When you work out, you want your heart rate to stay between those two numbers. Let's say you're fifty years old. 220 minus 50 is 170. That's your maximal heart rate. Multiply 170 by 0.6, and you get 102. Multiply 170 by 0.8, and you get 136. Your goal is to keep your heart rate between 102 and 136 while you work out.

What you will find is that the way my workouts are structured, it's hard not to have your heart rate in that range. The cardio portion will push it toward the higher end of the range, and during the weight lifting, it will fall toward, but generally not get lower than, the low end of the range.

You can always check for yourself. The same way you monitored your resting heart rate can be used to check your heart rate during your workout, with one exception. Since I don't want you stopping for an entire minute to do a heart rate check—that would let your heart rate drop lower than I want—you will check your pulse for only 10 seconds. Multiply that number by 6, and you'll have a good idea of your heart's beats per minute.

Extra-Credit Cardio

As I mentioned in the first chapter, if you want to do some extra cardio on the days when you're not doing one of my workouts, feel free. Unlike strength training, you can do cardio almost every day. Your body doesn't have to repair itself after you go for a jog or a swim. This is good and bad, and it shows you the specific benefits of cardio versus weight training. It's good because it means that you can walk, jog, bike, swim, and so on, a lot more often than you can lift weights. You can take advantage of the fact that you can quickly blaze through a whole lot of calories more frequently. The downside of cardio is that once you stop jogging or swimming and your heart rate returns to normal, you've stopped burning calories at an accelerated pace. With strength training, in addition to the calories you burn while you lift, your body spends the next 24 to 48 hours rebuilding the muscle that you've torn down while lifting weights. This rebuilding burns calories.

It's this difference between cardio and strength training that so few people understand. Most people who are trying to lose weight and firm up will do hours of cardio and maybe a few minutes of strength training. They look at the things they're doing in the weight room as being a complement to the work they're doing on the treadmill or the elliptical. The truth is, it's the other way around. Your cardio is really the complement to your strength training. Weight training is the prime mover in changing your body. Weight training causes your body to burn more calories around the clock than cardio does. Sure, you can look at a chart that says that weight lifting burns only 150 calories per hour compared to the 400 per hour that running does, but that's only a small part of the picture. Again, as soon as you finish your run, that 400-calories-per-hour meter inside you stops clicking and your body goes back to burning calories at its base metabolic rate. Strength training burns fewer calories per hour while you're in the weight room, but the real boost to your system is just beginning. Your body will spend the next two days burning calories at a higher rate while it repairs the muscles you've worked. And when the muscles are repaired, they will cause your body to burn more calories throughout the day. Cardio is a great tool, but it's not the be all and end all of getting in shape that most people think it is.

For us, the goal of cardio is to strengthen your cardiovascular system and serve as a turbo-boost to your calorie burning. Cardio enables you to burn a whole lot of calories in a short time. To ultimately get the results you're looking for, though, we need to make sure that what you lose is body fat and not muscle. Weight training will help you do that, but good nutrition—what you eat—will really ensure that your muscles are protected while your body fat is burned.

4

Celebrity Makeover Nutrition

Nutrition can be very difficult to understand, and there's no shortage of books and research studies on the subject. Some authors say one thing, and others say the exact opposite. You could go nuts trying to make heads or tails out of all the information and misinformation out there. But here's what I've found: I've trained thousands of clients and have been extremely successful with a proven program that I've developed. This nutrition program, coupled with my exercise program, will get you where you want to go faster than exercise or diet alone.

Hang with me, because once I give you the science behind my program, it'll all make sense. First off: eating fat will help you lose fat. Second: orange juice is one of the worst things you can have for breakfast. Third: bananas, corn, and certain vegetables can actually make you fat. So am I telling you to empty out the veggie bin in your fridge and fill it with bacon, sour cream, and mayo? No. Let me explain.

The food pyramid that we all learned as kids is a pretty flawed thing. The pyramids in Egypt have lasted for thousands of years, but the original food pyramid that was introduced to the world in 1974 has crumbled under the weight of scientific fact in less than forty years. It tells us to get most of our nutrients from breads, cereals, and pastas. It's a sound nutritional strategy only for people who've always dreamed of becoming obese.

The Glycemic Index

We now know that the glycemic index is the essential tool for losing weight, gaining weight, or simply maintaining weight. And it's not all that difficult to understand. The glycemic index was developed to rank foods according to their immediate effect on our blood-sugar levels.

If you've ever felt a temporary energy rush after eating a piece of chocolate, you've experienced a high blood-sugar level. And if you've ever sat at your desk at four-thirty in the afternoon, dead to the world and unable to lift a finger, you've experienced a low blood-sugar level. The key to weight management, as well as to energy management, is controlling your blood-sugar levels.

Carbohydrates that break down quickly during digestion have the highest glycemic value because the blood-sugar reaction is fast. Carbohydrates that break down more slowly, on the other hand, have a lower glycemic value because they enter the bloodstream at a far slower rate. The substance that triggers the greatest rise in blood-sugar levels is glucose itself. For that reason, pure glucose is rated as a perfect 100 out of 100 on the glycemic index. It's the Tiger Woods or Michael Jordan of sugars. Everything else is rated somewhere between 1 and 99, depending on its effect on the blood-sugar levels in our bodies.

Start your day with a doughnut and its glycemic value of 76, and you'll get a quick burst of energy, followed by a sluggish mid-morning hangover. Replace it with a slice of multigrain bread and its 48 glycemic value, and you'll have a consistent stream of energy that won't leave you drained by ten-thirty. Generally, the more processed a food is, the higher its glycemic value will be. That's why the doughnut—a yummy, deep-fried blend of processed white sugar and processed white flour—ranks so high, while the multigrain bread made from unprocessed grains ranks far lower.

How will this info help you shed the pounds? Contrary to what you may think, the fat in your diet isn't necessarily what's making you fat. The way your body deals with the excess carbs that you eat is what packs on the weight. Your body can handle only a certain amount of carbohydrates before it starts to convert all the extra carbs into body fat.

Even if your diet is relatively low in calories, if it's high in carbohydrates, you will have a tough time losing weight. As I'll explain, high levels of carbohydrates throw your entire system out of whack and prevent you from burning stored fat for energy. You might lose a few pounds initially, but eventually the weight loss ends. Meanwhile, you get more and more frustrated by the never-changing numbers on the scale and the fact that you're starving yourself and depriving yourself of the foods you like to eat. Eventually, you may throw up your hands and decide that you were never meant to be thin, glamorous, and sexy. Then you grab the nearest cheesecake. Game over. Six months later, you may try it again, but the same thing happens. Most of my new clients lived for years on this cycle of yo-yo dieting before I was able to help them out by explaining to them my simple, safe, and smart way to lose body fat.

The Truth about Carbs

So, carbs are the enemy? Not at all. Despite what some extreme diets suggest (and these are extreme diets that have been shown to be very unsuccessful in the long run), you need carbohydrates. Carbs are the only nutrients that feed the brain. If you're tired of having an active, productive, and healthy brain, then by all means stop eating your carbs. Carbohydrates are also your body's primary fuel for energy. The fact is, we need them, but we don't need an overabundance of them. Unfortunately, that's just what many people are eating.

Here's some more science: carbohydrates that aren't immediately used by the body get stored in the form of glycogen, which—in case you're ever a contestant on *Jeopardy*—is a series of glucose molecules strung together. The body has two beneficial storage areas for glycogen: the liver and the muscles. The brain can't access the glycogen stored in the muscles. It can use only the glycogen stored in the liver. The liver, though, has a very limited capacity to store a lot of glycogen. It can run dry in around ten to twelve hours. That's why we need to repeatedly eat carbohydrates. But what happens to the carbohydrates that we don't store in the liver or the muscles? They end up in a nonbeneficial storage area: our fat cells. And, again, that's our problem—not that we're eating carbs, but that we're eating way too many of them.

In addition to the number and the type of carbohydrates we eat, we also want to pay careful attention to when we eat them. When we eat carbs, our bodies release a hormone called insulin. Insulin is what grabs the carbs and brings them to the liver and the muscles. Think of insulin as being a bus. If we eat just a few carbs, out comes one of those little shopping mall shuttle buses to deliver the carbs to the liver and the muscles. Then it takes the few carbs that are left and puts them in the fat cells.

But what if we eat a lot of carbs? Now a fleet of buses—and I'm talking about the big double-decker sight-seeing ones—has to come out. As they all head to the fat cells, a traffic jam occurs. When insulin is present in our systems at those levels, we stop using our stored body fat as energy. If you eat before you work out, especially high-glycemic, high-carb meals or snacks, you'll never burn fat for energy because you've got too much insulin floating around in your system. None of that fat, or stored energy, that your body has squirreled away around your waist, butt, and thighs gets tapped into.

High levels of insulin in your system also affect and reduce the production of two other crucial hormones: glucagon and growth hormone. Glucagon promotes the burning of fat, which makes it a desirable thing to have around. Growth hormone is vital in the building of muscle, which is extremely important because increasing the amount of lean muscle on your body is one of the keys to my program. We can't afford to reduce the production of either of these hormones, but that's just what an increased level of insulin will do.

Consistently high levels of insulin have been linked to heart disease, diabetes, and hypertension. We want to send out as few buses as possible.

How do we eat carbs, as well as proteins and fats, optimally for weight loss? Fortunately, unless you have the palate of an eight-year-old and would happily exist on a steady diet of candy bars and soda, you're normally going to eat things other than carbs. Most of what we eat is composed of the three primary macronutrients: carbohydrates, proteins, and fats. You need all three of these nutrients, although not necessarily the same amount of each. Fats and protein, in addition to tasting good and satisfying your hunger, have the ability to reduce the glycemic value of the carbs that you eat. When you eat foods that are a combination of carbs, fats, and protein, your digestive system can't jump all over the simple sugars and pump them out into the bloodstream. It has to contend with the far-more-difficult-to-break-down proteins and fats at the same time. This delays the speed in which your blood-sugar level increases and, as a result, lowers the insulin response.

Of course, proteins and fats do more than that.

The Right Amount of Protein

While the main job of the carbs in your diet is to give you energy, the role of protein is to help build, maintain, and rebuild the cells of your muscles, organs, and so on. Proteins are composed of amino acids that are strung together like beads on a necklace. There are about two dozen different amino acids that your body uses to keep itself strong and healthy. They are building blocks that help to construct and repair your muscles. Your body can make all but nine of the amino acids. These nine are considered essential amino acids, which you have to get from your food. Proteins come from a variety of different sources: meat, fish, poultry, dairy, beans, and nuts. The proteins that we get from meat and dairy are considered complete proteins because they contain all of the essential amino acids. The proteins we get from vegetable sources are considered incomplete because they are missing one or more of the essential amino acids.

Don't worry, though, if you're trying to cut down on meat or are a vegetarian. Combining two incomplete proteins, such as rice and beans, can give you all the essential amino acids that you need. And you don't even have to eat them at the same time. As long as you have a varied diet, simply eating enough incomplete proteins will, at the end of the day, fulfill your body's requirement for these essential building blocks.

If your body needs to, it can even go through a process that converts proteins into carbohydrates that can be used for energy, but that's something you should keep to a minimum. You'll want to have the proper amount of carbohydrates in your diet so that your body doesn't have to tap into protein for energy. It's more efficient to use existing carbohydrates than to process them from proteins and, more important, carbohydrates are a heck of a lot cheaper. Think about it. Why fuel up on steak when you can do it more efficiently and less expensively with whole-grain bread?

The Right Kind of Fat

We need fat in our diet to help regulate our hormones and help us to better absorb nutrients from food. Fats can be broken down into four types, and, as you'll see, some are better for you than others are.

The Bad Fats

Saturated fats are generally fats that are solid at room temperature. Think about a stick of butter or the lines of white fat in a well-marbled piece of meat. Most saturated fat comes from animal or dairy products. A diet high in saturated fats has been shown to lead to high cholesterol levels and an increased risk of heart disease. When I describe my diet plan at the end of this chapter, you'll see that I try to steer you away from foods that are high in saturated fats.

Trans fats were first created by scientists in the early 1900s; and at the time they seemed like a really good thing. Food manufacturers used a process that turned liquid fats, such as oils, into solid fats like margarine by adding hydrogen. That's why you sometimes see trans fats referred to as "partially hydrogenated oils." Trans fats were designed to keep things fresher longer. Being realistic, if you baked a batch of crackers today, would you expect them to be edible a year from now? No, of course not. Baking with trans fats, as opposed to using a more perishable form of fat, such as oil, however, allows that box of crackers you bought at the store last week to virtually last forever. The drawback? Studies have shown that these trans fats might be even worse for us than saturated fats are when it comes to keeping our cholesterol levels in check. The rise in the rate of heart disease is truly scary since the introduction of trans fats into the modern food supply.

The Good News about Fat

Unsaturated fats can help you lower your cholesterol level and can decrease your chances of developing heart disease. Depending on their molecular structure, unsaturated fats fall into two categories: monounsaturated fats and polyunsaturated fats. These fats are unsaturated with hydrogen molecules that are eliminated in the forming of the fats' particular structure. The trans fats I previously talked about are unsaturated fats that are hydrogenated and, essentially, transformed into something resembling saturated fats. Hence the word *trans*.

Both monounsaturated fats and polyunsaturated fats have a liquid form at room temperature. Monounsaturated fats include and can be found in such things as nuts, olives, and avocados. Cooking with monounsaturated oils like olive oil, macadamia nut oil, and canola oil instead of butter is a great way to replace the heart-threatening fats in your diet with more heart-healthy fats.

You may have heard about the benefits of fish oil and how cultures that eat lots of fish have a far lower rate of heart disease. The reason for this is that fish oil is a particular type of polyunsaturated fat that contains omega-3 fatty acids. Studies have shown that diets that include fish oil not only lead to a decreased chance of developing heart disease, they can also promote a healthier brain, thanks to the omega-3 fatty acids' ability to help repair and grow brain cells. Do you want to have the smarts to go with your sexier new look? Eat more fish!

You should do your best to become a fish lover, but if you're not, don't worry. You can also get your omega-3s from flax. You can either buy whole flax seeds, crush them, and sprinkle them over yogurt or cereal or buy already-ground flaxseeds. Flaxseeds must be ground or your body can't access the fatty acids. The other alternative is to supplement your diet with flaxseed oil or fish oil. I'll talk more about supplements and vitamins at the end of the chapter.

Just as we need to limit the amount of carbs and protein we eat, we also have to keep an eye on the amount of fat we take in. Due to its composition, fat is the most calorically dense of the three macronutrients. A gram of protein has 4 calories. A gram of carbohydrates also has 4 calories. A gram of fat, though, has 9 calories. This means that gram-for-gram, fat has more than twice the number of calories of either protein or carbohydrates. For every gram of fat you remove from your diet, you can eat twice as much protein or carbs and still lose weight. Removing excess fat from your food is a great way to be able to eat more and still shed the pounds.

Eat Creatively, Eat Smartly

Happily, by using this knowledge of these three macronutrients, you can tweak the way that carbohydrates affect your blood-sugar levels. With some simple strategic tricks, you can drastically reduce the glycemic value of what you're eating to enable you to burn the most fat while you work out.

Here's a quick example. Say you're going to have an apple. It has a glycemic value of about 35 and contains around 60 calories. What if you cut the apple in half? Now you're looking at 30 calories. If you take a teaspoon of natural unsweetened no-salt peanut butter, which is around 30 calories, and put it on the apple, you're back up to a 60-calorie snack, but the protein and the fat in the peanut butter help to lower your body's sugar response to the carbs in the apple. The result is that you're taking in the same amount of calories, but your insulin response will be lower and you'll be eating something that—in my opinion—is much tastier than a plain old apple. You've used fat to help you lose fat, and you also added some bonus protein into your diet.

To make sure you keep your blood-sugar levels where they should be (and also eat enough to keep yourself happy), you ideally should be eating every two to three hours. By eating five or six times a day, you'll keep the amount you consume at any one time small enough for your digestive system to handle and you won't feel as if you're starving yourself. It's not the easiest schedule in world for some people to follow; life can sometimes get in the way. But if you're going to make a serious commitment to my program, this is how to get the most out it. You'll still have your three main meals, although they may end up being a little smaller than you're used to, but I've added three booster meals into the mix.

The benefit of having six small meals throughout the day is that this spaces out the food you eat and keeps your insulin response to a minimum by preventing your blood-sugar levels from getting too high. Just as important, it'll also keep your blood-sugar levels from dropping too low. When blood-sugar levels drop, you feel run down and start to crave sugar. This lethal combination easily results in your eating a whole mess of cookies. But by eating throughout the day, you'll have more energy than ever before, and you won't crave carbohydrates. Feel great while you lose weight? Imagine that.

Planning six meals a day can be much more difficult than planning three meals a day, but it's something you need to be able to do. I have my clients look at their schedule for the next day. If they're going to be home most of the day, that's great. Making sure they eat the right things at the right times will be easy. It's when they'll be out and about that they need to do some planning. Look at your schedule. If you're going to be out, you need to have something available that you can eat to keep your energy up and your blood-sugar levels in check. Some suggestions are a container of low-fat cottage cheese and an apple or a low-carb protein bar.

You may even find it helpful to plan out your entire week in advance. At the end of this chapter, I give you a full week's worth of meals and booster meals. Once you get past the initiation and introduction phases of the program (and more about those in a moment), you can use this menu in a couple of different ways: you could simply follow it for the remainder of the program and never have to think about what to eat, or you could use it as a template and personalize things by plugging in some of your favorite foods.

The night before you do your weekly shopping, pull out a piece of paper and, going day by day, come up with your three main meals and three booster meals. It's not as hard as it sounds, and you may be surprised at how creative you get. Feel free to use my sample menu for suggestions. Now, when you hit the supermarket, you'll know exactly what you need to get to keep you strong and energized for the week. By making sure that you have everything you need in the house, you'll be protecting yourself from the pitfalls that happen when you realize that it's time to eat and the only foods in the kitchen are crackers and ice cream.

Eventually, you may find yourself buying enough for the whole family to follow my plan. While your husband or wife may not be doing the exercise portion of the 30-Minute Celebrity Makeover Miracle, he or she will at least be able to benefit from the delicious and energy-boosting nutritional portion. Good nutrition, like fitness is general, is contagious. The key, though, is making sure you have everything you need. I can't overstate enough how important planning is. Without it, you're flying blind. It's like an actor showing up on the set without a script.

Proper nutrition is the key to success, and it all starts with breakfast. Bar none, breakfast is the most important meal of the day. Breakfast is just that: a breaking of a fast. You haven't eaten in nine or ten hours, and your body needs to be reminded that you love it and that you plan to feed it. As a survival mechanism left over from our caveman days, our bodies go into a starvation mode when food supplies are scarce and we haven't eaten for a while. This is why ultra-low-calorie diets don't work. Your body becomes very stingy with the way it burns calories and body fat. Eating breakfast gets your metabolism rolling so that you burn fat throughout the day.

"But wait," you say, "earlier, you said not to eat before I work out, and now you tell me that I need to eat breakfast. The only time I have to work out is first thing in the morning! Am I doomed? Should I go buy a different book?" Relax. While in a perfect world, you'd be able to wait an hour and a half after you ate before you exercised, I have some really good news for all of you early-morning types. The optimal time to eat protein is right after you've finished exercising. So, for those who can work out only in the morning, here's the fix: eat something small before you work out, such as an egg white omelet made with two egg whites, using nonstick spray instead of oil, or take a bite or two from a low-fat, low-carb protein bar. This will put something in your stomach so that your system will be happy, and because the food is virtually carb-free, it won't trigger much of an insulin response. After you exercise, you can eat some more protein to get the amino acids that will help to rebuild the muscle tissue. Your body also needs carbs after you exercise to replenish the glycogen stores that you depleted while you were sweating away.

The Makeover Miracle Nutrition Plan

How much protein should I eat? How many carbohydrates? How much fat? These are all good questions. I put my clients on a plan that works out to roughly 40 percent of their calories coming from protein, 40 percent from carbs, and 20 percent from fat. I've found that by sticking with a rough 40-40-20 formula, my clients lose weight without losing their minds. It's a very doable plan that your body won't have too many complaints with.

Some nutrition plans require you to weigh and measure every single item you put in your mouth. Sure, it would be nice to know that you're eating exactly 2.3 ounces of turkey, but is it really practical? You might be able to stay with that type of plan for about a day before you hurl the scale against the wall. Besides, if you carry a small scale around with you wherever you go, people will think that you're either a drug dealer or a really obsessive control freak. My plan doesn't require a scale. All you need is your hand. And since most people have two hands, at least one of them will usually be available.

I've made lists of primary and secondary proteins and carbs. Primary choices will be better for you. The proteins will be leaner, with a higher ratio of protein to fat. The carbs will be lower on the glycemic index. Secondary choices include protein sources that are a little bit fattier and carbs that may have a slightly higher glycemic value. Ideally, you'll stick to the primary choices as much as possible because it'll speed up the rate at which you reach your goals, and, as you'll soon see, you'll get to eat more food. Realistically, though, I don't expect anyone to survive on a steady stream of chicken breasts and nonfat cottage cheese. The secondary choices come in because, well, steak happens.

For each meal or booster meal, choose either a primary or a secondary protein and then break out your trusty hand. If your goal is to lose weight, the serving size of the protein should be the size of your palm. If you're happy with your weight but are looking to redistribute it on your body—in other words, to lose fat while you gain muscle—then the portion size should be your palm extended out to the first joint of your fingers. If you need to bulk up and want to make sure that you'll be adding muscle and not just fat, your portion size of protein should be the size of your entire hand.

Now, we go to my 1:2, 1:1, and 1:½ plan. And don't worry if you weren't all that good at math in school; this isn't difficult. If you choose a primary protein source, it can be either twice your protein portion's size of a primary carb or the same-size portion of a secondary carb. Let's say you're having salmon as your protein; you can have either a serving of green beans that's twice as big as the salmon (that's the 1:2 ratio) or a serving of pasta that's the same size (1:1). If you decide to eat a secondary protein, like the aforementioned steak, you can choose either a steak-size portion of a primary carb (1:1) or a half-portion-size serving of a secondary carb (1:½).

You may have noticed that there's no system for adding that 20 percent fat from my 40-40-20 plan into your diet. For the most part, we already get all the fat we need from the rest of our diet. And even though we will be eating fat to lose fat, there's generally no upside, except to the number on the scale, to adding butter or extra oil to the foods we eat.

Still hungry? I've also included a list of "free foods." These are foods that you can have one extra heaping serving of without their affecting your blood-sugar level or caloric intake all that much. They may not be the stuff of anyone's list of top ten foods of all-time. Has anyone ever really had a craving for celery? But they will help to keep you feeling full.

Here are the lists of primary and secondary proteins and carbs.

Primary Proteins

Chicken breast (fresh, not processed)

Cottage cheese (low-fat or nonfat)

Egg whites

Egg substitutes

Fat-free cheese

Fish (not processed)

Lean ground beef (15 percent fat or lower)

Hummus

Mock chicken or mock duck

Protein powder (whey for men, whey or soy for women)

Shellfish (any)

Soy burger

Soy hot dog

Soy sausage

Tempeh

Tofu

Turkey breast (fresh, not processed)

Secondary Proteins

All others—higher-fat cuts of red meat, dark meat poultry, and so on.

Primary Carbohydrates

Vegetables

Artichokes	Lentils
Asparagus	Lima beans
Bok choy	Mushrooms
Broccoli	Navy beans
Brussels sprouts	Pinto beans
Cabbage	Red beans
Cauliflower	Soybeans
Chickpeas	Spinach
Dried beans (any)	Squash
Green beans	Yams (baked)
Kale	Zucchini
Kidney beans	

Starches

Brown rice	Egg noodles

Cereals

Oatmeal, no sugar added	Unsweetened muesli with low-
Rolled oats	fat milk

Fruits

Apples	Peaches
Apricots (dried)	Pears
Berries	Plums
Cherries	Prunes
Grapefruit	Tomatoes
Oranges	

Dairy

Nonfat yogurt (with or without fruit) and sugar substitute

Secondary Carbohydrates

Vegetables

Beets	Parsnips
Carrots	Peas
Corn	Pumpkin

Starches, Cereals, and so on

Bread	Pretzels
Pasta	Puffed wheat
Popcorn	Rice (other than brown)
Potatoes	Rice cakes

Fruits

Applesauce	Kiwi fruit
Apricots	Honeydew
Bananas	Kumquats
Cantaloupe	Mango
Cranberries	Papaya
Dates	Pineapple
Figs	Raisins
Grapes	Watermelon

Free Foods

Bean sprouts	Jicama
Celery	Kale
Cucumber	Kohlrabi
Endive	Lemon juice
Fennel	Lettuce

Lime juice

Mushrooms

Mustard

Onions

Peppers

Radishes

Salsa

Sugar-free iced tea

Sugar-free instant cocoa

Sugar-free Jell-O

Sugar-free popsicles

Sugar-free sodas or other sugar-
free, nonfat drinks

Celebrity Nutrition Initiation and Introduction Phases

For the first two weeks of the program, you'll go through an initiation phase that'll kick-start your body into fat-burning mode. In the initiation phase, you're restricted to only primary proteins and carbs. You won't have as many options for what you get to eat, but you will be amazed at how fast you see results. The second two-week period is an introduction phase that'll ease you into my nutrition program. Here, half of all your meals and booster meals will be of the primary protein and primary carb variety. The other half can include secondary choices. It's still a limited version of my overall nutrition plan, but it's designed to let you continue to see positive results fast. For the final three phases of the program, when you burn the most calories and your body may need a little more energy, you'll be on the complete nutrition plan. I'll explain more about the initiation and introduction phases a little later.

As I mentioned earlier, you may want to add some dietary supplements into the mix. Remember, though, they're called supplements for a reason. They're intended to supplement the food you eat. The human body was designed to get its nutrients from the food it takes in. It's really good at doing this. This is how we survived as a species for so many millennia before the invention of chewable vitamins. If you're not a fish eater, you may want to add some fish oil to your diet. I recommend it in gel-cap form. You can go "old school" if you want to and take it straight in the form of cod liver oil, but be warned. You will be burping up a fishy taste for most of the day, and your breath might not be as sweet as you'd like.

A daily multivitamin is also a good idea. My nutrition plan does its best to make sure that you eat a wide variety of foods, but a multivitamin can be a good backup. I recommend a gender-specific vitamin. There are certain vitamins and minerals that women need more of than men do, and men need more of certain things than women do. A vitamin that takes this into account will ensure that you get what you need.

Eating right doesn't have to be as complicated as some people want you to think it is. So-called diet gurus and those infomercial folks hawking miracle weight-loss pills want you to believe that you're incapable of understanding proper nutrition so that you'll gladly hand over your credit card. The truth is that once you know the science behind how foods affect your body, it's relatively easy to make proper decisions for yourself.

Celebrity Makeover Sample Menu

To show you just how many different options you have, I've put together a week's worth of meals based on my nutrition plan. I've included three regular meals and three booster meals for each day. As you can see, not too many foods are off-limits. You'll still be able to have rice, pasta, corn, and so on. And to show you that eating well doesn't have to be boring, I've included meals that run the gamut from Italian and Mexican to Chinese and Japanese. My guess is that you'll be amazed at how well you'll be able to eat. You won't feel deprived, and you'll still lose weight and burn fat. If you want to, you can start with this menu on week five (after the initiation and introduction phases) and repeat it until the end of the program. Of course, you can also take any of the suggestions here and use them during the introduction phase. If you love to cook and want to be creative, or if I've listed some foods that you aren't too fond of, feel free to swap in whatever you want. Just make sure you replace a primary protein or carb with a primary protein or carb and secondary proteins and carbs with secondary proteins and carbs. Bon appetit!

Sunday

Breakfast	Oatmeal and a cup of low-fat milk
Booster Meal #1	Pear with 2 ounces hummus
Lunch	Salmon over salad greens, topped with one tablespoon of salsa
Booster Meal #2	Half grapefruit and ten no-salt cashews
Dinner	Chicken stir-fry (using a nonstick spray instead of oil) over a small amount of egg noodles, along with a green salad topped with fresh-squeezed lemon or lime juice
Booster Meal #3	Cherries and nonfat yogurt topped with no-sugar-added, low-fat whipped cream

Monday

Breakfast	Low-fat yogurt—½ cup
Booster Meal #1	Ten raw almonds and a medium orange
Lunch	Turkey breast, a small amount of corn, a green salad topped with one tablespoon of salsa, and six cherries
Booster Meal #2	One tomato cut into wedges dipped in hummus
Dinner	One meatball in marinara sauce over a small amount of spaghetti, along with a green salad topped with one tablespoon of salsa
Booster Meal #3	A small handful of salt-free peanuts

Breakfast	Three egg whites with mixed vegetables (You can sauté everything together using a nonstick spray instead of oil.)
Booster Meal #1	Low-fat protein bar
Lunch	Broccoli and zucchini over a small amount of brown rice, a salad topped with one tablespoon of salsa, and a protein shake. (This is an example of a vegetarian option.)
Booster Meal #2	Tomato slices topped with a small amount of part-skim buffalo mozzarella
Dinner	Chicken kebab and a small amount of brown rice, along with a mixed green salad topped with one tablespoon of salsa
Booster Meal #3	Pear with one tablespoon of low-fat peanut butter

Wednesday

Breakfast	Low-fat or nonfat cottage cheese with a half-cup of berries
Booster Meal #1	Three celery sticks with 1 ounce of low-fat peanut butter
Lunch	Sashimi, miso soup, soybeans (edamame), and a mixed green salad topped with a combination of soy sauce and vinegar
Booster Meal #2	Fruit salad and low-fat yogurt
Dinner	Small lean cut of steak, peas, and a small amount of baked beans, along with a green salad topped with a sliver of avocado and slivers of grapefruit

Booster Meal #3	Strawberries and nonfat yogurt topped with no-sugar-added, low-fat whipped cream

Thursday

Breakfast	Three egg whites and a grapefruit
Booster Meal #1	1 ounce of skim milk cheese (or any nonfat cheese) and a medium apple
Lunch	Chicken breast, broccoli, and lentils, along with a mixed green salad topped with one tablespoon of salsa
Booster Meal #2	Low-fat, low-carbohydrate protein bar
Dinner	Grilled ahi tuna steak and half a palm-sized serving of broccoli, along with a green salad topped with one tablespoon of salsa. For dessert, one scoop of no-sugar-added ice cream. (This is an example of how you can have ice cream for dessert. What we did was take a primary carb and cut it in half. The carbs you saved during dinner can then be eaten as your dessert. This isn't the way I want you to eat on a regular basis—broccoli is a lot better for you than ice cream is—but it shows how you can still have dessert every once in a while.)
Booster Meal #3	Ten raw cashews and a large plum

Friday

Breakfast	Low-fat yogurt and a half-cup of berries
Booster Meal #1	Peel-and-eat shrimp with a salsa dip

Lunch	Chicken breast mixed with egg pasta, along with a green salad topped with one tablespoon of salsa
Booster Meal #2	Low-fat, low-carb protein shake
Dinner	Small pita pizza made with tomato sauce, mushrooms, bell peppers, or any vegetables in the primary carb list, topped with low-fat mozzarella cheese (if you don't want cheese, feel free to substitute chicken or any other primary protein)
Booster Meal #3	Fruit smoothie made with ¼ cup of berries blended with nonfat, no-sugar-added yogurt

Saturday

Breakfast	Granola with 1 cup of low-fat milk
Booster Meal #1	Medium apple and one tablespoon of peanut butter
Lunch	Shrimp, grapefruit sections, and five sliced almonds over mixed greens, topped with one tablespoon of salsa
Booster Meal #2	Fruit salad and low-fat yogurt
Dinner	Grilled salmon, lentils, and a baked yam, along with a green salad topped with fresh-squeezed lemon or lime juice
Booster Meal #3	I saved the best for last—my famous protein pudding. Take Jell-O sugar-free pudding mix and 1 scoop of your favorite low-fat, low-carb protein powder. Mix them dry, then add low-fat milk or lactose-free, low-fat milk. Chill as instructed on the pudding package. Then have a full palm's worth of this protein treat.

Celebrity Makeover Tips and Tricks

Actors and actresses have no shortage of tricks they use to help them memorize their lines and get into character. When it comes to staying on the 30-Minute Celebrity Makeover Miracle nutrition plan, there are also some cool tips, tricks, and bits of advice that will help you be successful. These aren't cheats or shortcuts. They're just little things you can do to make sure that you're eating right and sticking to my plan.

If you eat out a lot, don't be afraid to ask for substitutions. Request extra vegetables (ideally steamed) instead of rice, pasta, or a potato. As long as you're nice about it, most restaurants won't mind. They want your business. When you first sit down in a restaurant, have the waiter or the waitress remove the breadbasket from the table. There's no faster way to overload on carbs and calories, and completely sabotage my nutrition program, than by starting your meal off with a hunk or two of unneeded bread.

If you eat in front of the TV, always have a premeasured amount of food. I don't care who you are or what you say, if you sit down in front of the TV with a jar of peanuts and tell me that you're only going to eat ten of them, you're living in a fantasy world.

Always have a backup plan. If the banana that you were going to eat for your mid-morning booster meal didn't survive the overcrowded train ride into work, make sure that you have a low-fat, low-carb protein bar in your desk. A backup plan reduces your chances of heading to the candy machine for a snack.

Store pre-measured amounts of food in plastic bags. If you do a lot of running around, it's a great way to make sure that you'll not only have the right foods to eat but that you're eating the proper amount. A handful of raisins tossed in a bag with a few almonds or a couple of apple wedges topped with no-salt peanut butter will give you just the protein and carbohydrates you need. If you've never met a bag of raisins or a jar of peanut butter that you haven't been tempted to finish, these pre-measured portions are a godsend.

Brush your teeth after dinner and before dessert is offered. If you have a clean, fresh-tasting mouth, you'll be less likely to give in to sweets that can sabotage your nutrition plan. Can't brush? Chewing on a piece of sugar-free gum can have the same result.

Drinking Do's and Don'ts

Drink plenty of water. Aim for eight glasses (64 ounces) every day. Not only will it guarantee that you stay hydrated, which is especially important since you're involved in a fitness program, it will also keep you feeling full and less hungry during the day.

Drink a glass of room-temperature water first thing in the morning. It will help to fill you up and get you started on a pace for eight glasses. The fact that the water is room temperature is important because it won't shock your system.

Drink water with meals. You'll feel fuller without adding any extra calories or carbs to your meal.

Avoid alcohol with meals. If you want a drink—one drink!—count it as your serving of carbs for the meal.

Alcohol does more than just put empty calories into your body. It can also cause you to let down your guard. The reason I want you to stop at one drink with dinner is that two or more drinks often leads to an order of french fries and chocolate mousse for dessert.

Avoid caffeine in the evening. Anything that cuts into the amount or the quality of your sleep takes away from my program. Your body does a lot of its muscle-building repair work while you sleep. You also have to be well-rested enough to give it your all while working out. If you're a big coffee drinker, try switching to green tea. It's lower in caffeine than coffee is, so you won't go into caffeine withdrawal, as you might if you switch straight to decaf. Green tea is also loaded with antioxidants.

Common Mistakes

Vacation calories do count! Just because you're away from home and away from work, it doesn't mean all bets are off when it comes to eating. You may be on vacation, but for your heart, lungs, muscles, and metabolism, it's business as usual. Staying on a nutrition plan when you're traveling can be difficult. You're out of your element. There are more temptations. If you're staying in a hotel room that doesn't have a refrigerator, you're forced to eat just about all of your meals in restaurants. You don't have to suffer, though. In fact, I want you to splurge. Instead of splurging on quantity, I want you to splurge on quality. You could eat a lot of pretty good food and fall off of your nutrition plan, or you could spend a little bit more—you are on vacation after all—and get a lesser amount of *really* good food. What could be better than the best fish or seafood you can find in San Francisco or Boston, or the best cut of lean beef you can get in Kansas City? Eating smaller portions of high-quality food will keep you on your plan (and keep your energy levels up while you travel) and it will also give you culinary memories that will last a lifetime.

Avoid buffets. No phrase has done more to undermine the health and fitness of Americans than "all you can eat." Whether it's on a flashing neon sign by the side of the road or it's been neatly hand-scripted on a chalkboard outside a quaint family restaurant, stay away! It's been hammered into our heads since we were children that we need to get our money's worth, that money doesn't grow on trees, and that we can't leave food on our plates because there are starving people in the world. All-you-can-eat buffets prey on all of these drummed-in concepts. You're almost being challenged from the get-go to eat more than you really want and to clean your plate. Restaurateurs are more than happy to see you filling you plate again and again. They're glad that you think you're getting even more than your money's worth. The way they make money is by serving up very inexpensive foods in huge quantities. And inexpensive food, generally, isn't all that high in nutritional value.

Even so-called healthy buffets may not be all they're cracked up to be. Take the "egg bar," for example. You could get a high-protein, low-carb egg-white omelet made fresh right in front of you, but if you look at how it's being cooked, it's swimming in a half-inch of butter and oil. This potentially heart-healthy and muscle-friendly meal has been reduced to a high-fat, high-calorie heart risk. All-you-can-eat sushi is another trap. People think that sushi is good for you. It is, but not if you consume the equivalent of your body weight of it. Most of what you eat when you eat sushi is rice. Due to the way sushi rice is prepared, it's not only been stripped of most of its nutritional value, but it's been sweetened with sugared vinegar. You end up eating far too much of very high-glycemic carbohydrates.

Don't drink your calories. A major trap that people fall into is that they don't think about all the calories that are in the things they drink. I have no problem with coffee, for example, in limited amounts. It can be a great pick-me-up, but all coffee drinks are not created equally. If you take a 16-ounce cup of coffee and add a packet of artificial sweetener like Splenda and a little bit of skim or 1% milk, you're fine. It's a very low-calorie, low- or zero-fat drink. On the other hand, if you think that "coffee is coffee," your system will be in for a shock. If you chose a blended drink, like one of those caramel frappuccino things, you may unwittingly be pouring 400 calories and 15 grams of fat into your body.

Fruit juices are another pitfall. Everyone assumes that because something's all natural and made from real fruit, it must be good for you. An 8-ounce glass of orange or apple juice can have as many as 28 grams of sugar. That's 28 grams of high-glycemic carbs. The label may say "fat-free," but that can be misleading. Remember, high-glycemic carbs cause an insulin response that tells your body to store excess carbs as fat. That "fat-free" on the label refers only to the juice going into your system. Once it's in, it's a different story.

By the way, do you want to know what 28 grams of sugar look like? A teaspoon of sugar is 16 calories. If you remember that when I talked about the differences between fats, proteins, and carbohydrates, I told you that a gram of carbohydrate contained 4 calories.

That means that a teaspoon of sugar is 4 grams; 28 grams would be 7 teaspoons of sugar. The next time you're in your kitchen, put 7 teaspoons of sugar in a glass. That's the amount of sugar in your orange juice. Now pour in 7 ounces of water. That'll bring things up to 8 ounces. Give it a stir. I know, it's not dissolving all that well. Now take a sip. That's what your body deals with when you drink fruit juice. Your body isn't soaking up Florida sunshine; it's getting flooded with too much sugar.

Another nutrition trap we fall into is not understanding food labels. The FDA has done a wonderful job of making sure that the foods we buy are properly labeled. We now know what the exact ingredients are, the number of calories, and how many grams and micrograms of protein, carbohydrates, fats, vitamins, and minerals there are. It's a luxury that our parents and grandparents didn't enjoy. For people with severe allergies, just the ingredients list alone can literally be a lifesaver. That said, I find that many people don't read these labels carefully enough.

I purposely don't include a lot of calorie and fat-gram counting in my nutritional plan, but that doesn't mean you should be unaware of what you're eating. I find the biggest mistake people make is when it comes to serving size. A package of "diet" potato chips may say that it has only 70 calories and 1 gram of fat. It's not the greatest thing you can eat, but it's not the worst. The problem is that after you've eaten the entire bag, you realize that the bag contained six servings. Now you have to multiply your figures by 6, and all of a sudden, you've taken in too many calories and fat. Manufacturers are very good at making the numbers on the nutrition information label look deceptively healthy.

5

Getting Started

In a short while, I'm going to ask you to put this book down and think about a few things. Think about the way you look now and, just as important, the way you feel about the way you look. Now think about the next ten weeks. Literally, picture the days as they appear on the calendar or in your appointment book. Picture the calendar pages being turned or ripped away as the months change. Picture the weather changing outside as the seasons progress. Picture the way your backyard or your neighborhood will look in ten weeks. Will the grass be greener? Will the leaves be turning colors? What will the air smell like? Then, I want you to envision a new you walking around in that ten-weeks-from-now world. A leaner you. A stronger you. A more confident you. Think about how you'll feel in your new body and about how others will feel about you and your new body.

Now, put down the book, close your eyes, and think—really think—about how different your life can be in just ten weeks. Take your time. I'll still be here when you're done.

What did you feel? If you felt a jolt of excitement and adrenaline, that's the same feeling I get whenever I start with a new client. It's the excitement of knowing just how profoundly better someone will look and feel in the near future. Ten weeks is not a long time. I'm giving you everything you need to transform your body and your life over the next ten weeks, but if it's going to work, you have to commit yourself to it. Just as with my clients, this is a partnership. I'm in this with you. I'm giving you my knowledge, experience, and guidance. In return, I need a promise of commitment from you.

Here's what that means. You are going to work out three times a week. It can be Monday, Wednesday, and Friday. It can be Tuesday, Thursday, and Saturday. But it needs to be three times per week, every week, with a day's rest between workouts. To make this happen and to really change your body, you have to make working out a priority. Even when time gets tight, you have to set aside that half-hour for your workout. That's all I'm asking for. It has to become a mandatory part of your day, like showering or brushing your teeth.

Here's what you'll need for the program:

- A stability ball. Use a 45-centimeter ball if you're five feet, two inches, or shorter, or a 55-centimeter ball if you're taller.

- Three or four pairs of dumbbells. If you're a woman, they should range from 3 to 10 pounds. If you're a man, they should range from 5 to 20 pounds. They must be in pairs; mismatched dumbbells won't work.

- A comfortable pair of cross-training athletic shoes.

- Comfortable clothes to exercise in.

- An easy-to-read clock with a second hand.

As you can see, the 30-Minute Celebrity Makeover Miracle does not require you to go out and buy a lot of expensive equipment, and you're not going to have to give up a room in your house just to store the stuff. You'll be amazed at what you are going to accomplish with just a few dumbbells and a stability ball, and when you're finished working out, you'll be equally amazed at how little space your home gym takes up. Most everything can be picked up at your local sporting goods store, but if you are having trouble finding anything, I've enclosed a list of online stores at the end of the book that carry everything you'll need.

Track Your Progress

Before we begin, let's get a snapshot of where you are now. While the ultimate goal of the 30-Minute Celebrity Makeover Miracle is to dramatically change the way you look and feel, it never hurts to be able to back up your results with a little raw data.

First, I want you to take some body measurements. I want you to measure and write down the dimensions of your chest, waist, neck, shoulders, and hips and your right and left biceps (when flexed), thighs, and calves.

Use the worksheet on page 75 to fill in your initial measurements. I've included worksheets at the end of each two-week phase of the 30-Minute Celebrity Makeover Miracle to let you monitor where you are losing fat, gaining muscle, and so on.

Check Your Body Fat Percentage

To see just how much fat you'll be losing, we're going to do a body fat analysis. Ideally, you could go to a pricey, elite training facility and have them measure the percentage of your total weight that is fat. Unfortunately, that could cost thousands of dollars. For our purposes, we'll use a much less expensive method. It's free, actually. It will give you a reasonably accurate idea of where you stand. All you'll need is a calculator, unless you're really good at math.

Women

1. Step on the scale and weigh yourself.

   Your body weight (in pounds) _____ $\times 0.732 + 8.987 =$ _____

2. Measure your wrist at the fullest point.

   Your wrist measurement (in inches) _____ $\div 3.140 =$ _____

3. Measure your waist at your navel.

   Your waist measurement (in inches) _____ $\times 0.157 =$ _____

4. Measure your hips at the fullest point.

   Your hips measurement (in inches) _____ × 0.249 = _____

5. Measure your forearm at the fullest point.

   Your forearm measurement (in inches) _____ × 0.434 = _____

To calculate your body fat:

   Add the totals for 1 and 2.

   Subtract the total for 3.

   Subtract the total for 4.

   Add the total for 5.

This is your lean body mass (muscle, bones, organs, hair, and so on) in pounds.

   Subtract your lean body mass from your total weight.

   Total body weight (in pounds) _____ − lean body mass _____ = _____ pounds

This is the weight of your body fat.

Multiply your body fat weight by 100, then divide by your total body weight.

   Body fat weight _____ × 100 = _____ ÷ total body weight = _____ percent

This is your body fat percentage.

Men

1. Step on the scale and weigh yourself.

   Your body weight (in pounds) _____ × 1.082 + 94.42 = _____

2. Measure your waist.

   Your waist measurement (in inches) _____ × 4.15 = _____

To calculate your body fat:

   Subtract the total of 2 from the total of 1.

   Measurement 1 _____ − measurement 2 _____ = _____ pounds

This is your lean body mass in pounds.

Subtract your lean body mass from your total weight.

Total body weight _____ (in pounds) – lean body mass _____

= _____ pounds

This is the weight of your body fat.

Body fat weight (in pounds) _____ × 100 = _____ ÷ total body

weight = _____ percent

This is your body fat percentage.

So what do all those fancy calculations tell you? The following chart will help you figure out where you stand right now in terms of body fat percentage:

Level	Men	Women
Excellent	<12	<18
Good	12–16	18–20
Acceptable	17–20	21–25
Fair	21–23	26–29
Unacceptable	24+	30+

Notice that I had two separate formulas for determining body fat percentage, one for men and one for women. The chart also breaks down the results by gender, because women are built differently from men. They generally carry a higher percentage of weight and fat around the chest and hips. The formulas take that into account and so does the chart. A body fat percentage of 18 on a woman is considered excellent, but that same percentage on a man is considered only acceptable.

Don't be upset if your current percentage level isn't as good as you expected. This is your initial reading. You have nowhere to go but up (or, actually, down). Your body fat percentage, along with the measurements you'll be taking of your chest, waist, hips, biceps, and so on, will give you a solid read on how much progress you're making on the 30-Minute Celebrity Makeover Miracle. They give you a far greater barometer of how fit you're becoming than a lone number on the bathroom scale does.

Say you're a 200-pound man with a body fat percentage of 25 percent. A quarter of your weight, or 50 pounds, is fat. This puts you in the unacceptable category. Now you start to work out. You go through the walking phase and the marching phase, and you're feeling great. If you stepped on the scale, there's a good chance that the number may still say 200. "How is that possible?" you ask as you angrily rifle through your files, looking for the receipt for this book so that you can get your money back.

In the 4 weeks that it took you to make it through the walking and marching phases, you've burned a ton of calories and burned a whole lot of fat. You've also built a lot of lean muscle. That was our plan. You did your cardio to burn calories and your strength training to build metabolism-boosting muscle. There's a good chance that while you may have burned off a full 15 pounds of fat, you could have built 15 pounds of muscle. On the scale, it appears that you're exactly the same as when you started, but now let's look at the body fat percentage numbers. If you walked and marched away 15 pounds of fat, you now are carrying only 35 pounds of fat on your body. That's a body fat percentage of just 17.5 percent. On the chart, that puts you right on the border of good and acceptable. Not a bad leap from unacceptable.

This decrease in body fat percentage isn't just a number on a chart in a book, though. While your scale may still say 200, you've replaced 15 pounds of fat with 15 pounds of muscle. Muscle is a lot more dense than fat. A pound of muscle takes up a lot less space than a pound of fat. If you replace 15 pounds of fat with 15 pounds of lean and sexy muscle, you'll physically be smaller. Your muscles will appear more defined and your clothes will fit differently. They'll be a lot looser around the stomach, hips, and wherever else your body was storing fat. Your friends and coworkers will ask you if you've lost weight. My bet is that if you tell them the truth and say that you haven't, they'll just think you're being modest. Too many people obsess over the number on the scale. The fact is that it's just one of many ways to track your progress.

Every two weeks, at the start of each new workout phase, you'll recheck all of your numbers. This will let you track your progress and will give you the hard facts behind the hard body that you see shaping up, day by day, in the mirror before you.

Get Ready Mentally

All right. We've gone through the science and the theories behind the program. You've taken your measurements, and you're ready to see them dramatically altered. You have all the equipment you need. Physically, you're ready to go. One last thing: we have to get you ready mentally. It's just as important to be mentally prepared to exercise as it is to be physically prepared. Your mood, the way you feel—your mental state—can make or break a workout. It's the difference between feeling supercharged, in the zone, and feeling tired, sluggish, and distracted. Your head has to be in the workout as much as your body does.

The night before every workout, look at the exercises that you'll be doing. I want you to do this for two reasons. First, it will give you a chance to review the proper technique for the exercises so that there won't be any interruptions during the workout. Second, it'll prepare you mentally and let you focus on what you have to do.

The Cleansing Minute

Just before every workout, turn off your cell phone and turn down the ringer on your house phone. If there's a TV blaring in the next room, turn it off. Put on music you like and that motivates you. It can be anything you want—classical, hip-hop, show tunes, anything—as long as it will keep you going.

As you run down the list of workouts you'll do, you'll see that the first item on every workout is a "cleansing minute." Even though I've talked about the importance of moving your body and keeping it moving, you're going to spend the first minute of every workout almost motionless. You'll spend a minute cleansing your mind of outside thoughts and distractions and focusing on your body and your workout.

Imagine a circle about three feet in diameter on the floor. Now, step inside the circle. For the next 30 minutes, concentrate only on what's inside that circle—namely, you. Nothing outside the circle matters, not the dog, the cat, the neighbors, the score of last night's game, your aunt's recent knee surgery. Close your eyes, and take a deep breath. Inhale through the nose and exhale through the mouth. Take three deep breaths this way. Forget about your hectic schedule and the things you have to do. Any worries that you have in your mind right now will still be there in 30 minutes. Push them aside for half an hour. The next 30 minutes are all about you. For maybe the only block of time in your entire day, you have to make yourself the most important person in your life.

Take another deep breath and exhale. Feel your body. Wiggle your toes and fingers. Rotate your ankles and wrists. Slowly bounce and feel your knees, hips, elbows, and shoulders. Feel your muscles and joints. Concentrate on them. They are the tools and the weapons that you will need for the next half-hour. Talk to them if you have to: "Get ready, legs, shoulders, and arms. We have work to do." Get them on your side. Think of your entire body as a team.

Now, go back and review the things I told you to think about at the beginning of the chapter: how you feel about the way you look, the calendar changing as ten weeks goes by, how your neighborhood will look at the end of the program, how you will look at the end of the program, how good you'll feel at the end of the program. Finally, picture yourself blazing confidently through your workout, feeling your muscles, your bones, your heart, your lungs, and your entire body getting stronger. Picture yourself alive and full of energy. Picture yourself finishing your workout and not being able to wait until you can do it all again. Visualize it. Take another deep breath, exhale slowly, and open your eyes.

You're just ten weeks away from a new you.

Getting Started Worksheet

Initial Measurements

Neck _____ Shoulders _____

Chest _____ Waist _____ Hips _____

Right biceps (flexed) _____ Left biceps (flexed) _____

Right thigh _____ Left thigh _____

Right calf _____ Left calf _____

Resting heart rate _____

Body fat percentage _____

6

Celebrity Makeover Exercises

I'm now going to introduce you to the strength-training exercises that you'll be doing. I'll do more than just give you a list of things to do and set you loose. I'll explain the science and the philosophy behind the movements. I want you to understand why you're doing something and how your body works. It's like that old adage: give a man a fish and he eats for a day; teach a man to fish and he eats for a lifetime. (I also like that adage for another reason: because it will remind you to eat plenty of healthy, high-protein, brain-boosting fish.) I don't want to merely give you a workout to follow; I want to teach you the concepts behind the workout so that you can see the logic of what you're doing. Then you'll eventually be able to come up with workout variations on your own that are just as balanced and carefully thought out as the ones I've given you.

I've broken the exercises down into sections: the chest, the back, the shoulders, the arms, the lower body (butt, thighs, and calves), and the abs. For each body part, I've given an explanation of what our goals are in developing and strengthening that area. For women and men, the goals can often be very different. I've also explained how the individual muscles actually work. It's not heavy-duty science, but it's enough to give you a big picture view of the human body. Once you understand the mechanics of how the body moves, it'll be that much easier to make sure you get the most from each exercise. Then you'll see better results and be more excited about your next workout.

Every exercise includes photographs that show you the key positions of the exercise and provide a detailed description of the proper technique. I want things to be crystal clear for you, so that when you work out, your mind is focused on getting the most out of your body instead of wondering whether you're doing the exercise correctly. Because the goal of my program is to keep your heart rate up throughout the entire workout and avoid any downtime, it's a good idea to familiarize yourself with the exercises you'll be doing before the actual workout starts. My advice is to take a couple of minutes at the end of your workout to see what you'll be doing for your next workout. This has two benefits. First, you can review the technique for an exercise you may not have done for a while or practice the form for a new one. Second, you can start doing that mental visualization I talked about. If you have a full forty-eight hours to get mentally prepared for a workout, trust me, you'll be able to blaze through it when the time comes.

A lot of the exercises also have information that's specific to each movement. The comments can be about anything, from how a certain wrist or grip position can affect the outcome of an exercise to the various do's and don'ts of a technique. Read these comments. Along with the information about the individual muscles, they help to make this chapter a user's manual for the human body. And since you've had the good fortune to be blessed with a human body, the more you know about it, the better.

As I mentioned in chapter 2, "Strength," there may be times when you'll have trouble getting the technique down for a certain exercise. If you have a problem with a particular exercise, seeing the exercises grouped by body part will allow you to easily make a substitution that will still develop and strengthen that same muscle group.

These exercises are the main tools you'll use to transform your body. They are the same exercises I use with my celebrity clients to get them looking and feeling their best. I've chosen them carefully to let you see the results you want, quickly.

Celebrity Upper Body

The perfect upper body is a classic case of the whole being greater than the sum of its parts. The individual players (the chest, back, shoulders, and arms) need to look their best, but when you bring them all together, each part makes those around it shine even brighter. For both men and women, the goal is a strong posture and a V-shaped torso that tapers down to a trim waist. Men will have a more pronounced V-shape. Their shoulders will be wider than their hips. Women will have a narrower V-shape, with shoulders being equal in size to their hips. Now that you understand the goal, let's break it down and show you how it's going to happen.

Celebrity Chest

A well- and properly developed chest is a vital part of the celebrity look. Whether you're a woman or a man, a strong chest announces your presence. It implies confidence. When we want to impress or intimidate someone, we stick out our chests without even realizing it. The sex appeal of both sexes is intimately related to the chest.

A properly developed chest doesn't happen by accident, though. The chest muscles have to be built up in a strategic way. For women, the goal is to work the upper part of the muscle. Developing this area will lift the breasts, giving you a more youthful look. For women, developing the chest correctly can almost mimic the results of cosmetic breast surgery.

For men, developing the chest involves slightly more finesse. If you work as a lifeguard or a topless dancer, you might be able to get away with a bodybuilder's chest and those huge bowling ball–sized chest muscles. Unfortunately, though, most of us have to wear clothes. The problem with a giant chest is that unless you can have every shirt you own custom-tailored, a lot of the time you'll end up looking fat. The key for men to properly developing the chest is in figuring out where to add size and where to do some sculpting. The actor Vin Diesel doesn't have an Arnold-like chest, but that doesn't make his chest any less enviable. The key to his look is that he worked to add size to the upper part of the chest. This gives the whole muscle an even and proportioned look. Developing only the middle or the lower part of the chest can give you a saggy appearance. The other keys are the clear separation between the left and the right chest muscles and the sculpting of the outer edge of the muscles. It's these delineations that give him a cut, sculpted, athletic look—a look that implies strength and virility.

Chest Muscles

The pectoralis major is the large muscle that runs from your armpit to the center of your chest, just below your collarbone, and then down to the middle of your rib cage. Your pecs have a few different jobs. Mainly, they're the primary muscles used in pushing motions. Every time you push open a door or push a lawn mower, you're using your pecs. These pressing motions are the main way that you add size to the pecs. If you were using heavy dumbbells or barbells, you'd be adding lots of size, but since your goal is tone and the proper distribution of size, all of your pressing motions are push-up-based, using just your own body weight. The muscle's other function is to draw your arm inward from an outstretched position. Stand with your arms out to the sides, as if you're making a giant letter T. Keeping your arms straight and your elbows from bending, slowly clap your hands in front of you at shoulder height. That was your pecs at work. This movement really develops the separation between the left and the right pec, and it's essentially the same motion that you'll do in both the Hollywood Fly and the Hollywood Incline Fly.

Beginner Push-Up

The push-up is almost the perfect exercise. It works the chest, the triceps, the shoulders, the abs, and the lower back and doesn't require even a dollar's worth of equipment. This is a starter push-up. As your upper body gets stronger, you'll be able to advance to the more challenging variations.

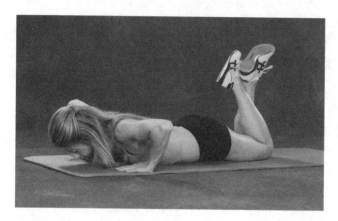

GET READY

Lie facedown on the floor and bend your knees behind you, lifting your feet off the floor. Cross your ankles. Place your palms on the floor, slightly wider than shoulder-width apart, at chest level.

DO THE EXERCISE

Take a deep breath. Pull your belly button in and exhale and press away from the floor so that you're balancing on your hands and knees. Keep your body rigid, so that there's a straight line running from your knees to the top of your head. Hold for a beat, and inhale as you lower yourself toward the floor. Avoid letting your chest touch the floor in this lowered position. Hold for a beat, exhale, and repeat.

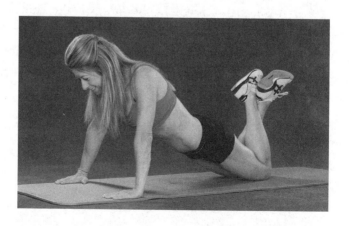

Intermediate Push-Up

This is the same as the Beginner Push-Up but military-style. Instead of supporting yourself on your knees, you'll be up on your toes.

GET READY
Lie facedown on the floor with your toes curled under your feet. Place your palms on the floor, slightly wider than shoulder-width apart, at chest level.

DO THE EXERCISE
Take a deep breath. Exhale and press your body away from the floor until you're balanced on your hands and toes. Again, you want your body to be in a straight line, so avoid letting your butt rise up in the air. Hold this up position for a beat and slowly lower yourself almost to the floor as you inhale. Hold this down position for a beat, and repeat.

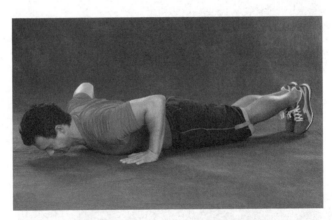

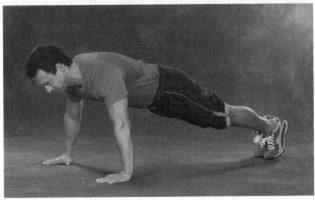

Advanced Push-Up

This one is a challenge, but with a few tweaks, you can make it easier to get used to. The placement of the ball in relation to your body greatly affects the difficulty of the push-up. Move the ball higher up on your body—under your hips, for example—to make things a little easier. If you want to ramp things up, slide the ball lower on your body so that only your feet are on the ball, to make it even tougher.

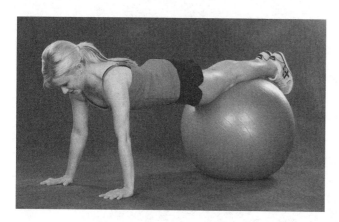

GET READY

Drape yourself facedown over a stability ball and walk your hands forward until the ball is resting under your thighs. Lock your elbows so that your arms are straight. They should be at chest level and slightly wider than shoulder-width apart. Just as with the beginner and the advanced push-up, keep your body in a straight line throughout the exercise.

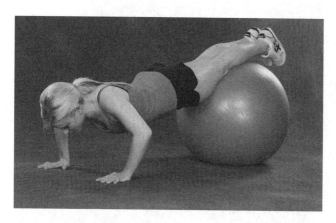

DO THE EXERCISE

Inhale as you slowly lower your chest to within an inch or two of the floor, keeping your body straight as you go. Hold this down position for a beat, then press yourself back up to the starting position as you exhale. Hold for a beat, then repeat.

Hollywood Fly

This is a great way to sculpt the edges of your pecs. You can almost feel your pecs getting larger as you squeeze them together at the top of this motion.

GET READY
Lie back on a stability ball so that the ball is under the upper part of your back and your head is well-supported in a natural position. Your chin shouldn't be jammed into your chest, and your head shouldn't hang off the ball. Place the tip of your tongue behind your top front teeth. Position your feet directly under your knees, about hip-width apart. Push your hips up so that there's a straight and parallel line running from your knees to your shoulders. With a dumbbell in each hand, palms facing up, extend your arms out to either side with your elbows bent and pointed downward.

DO THE EXERCISE
Take a deep breath. Exhale and drive the weights upward as if you were hugging a stability ball. At around the halfway point, slowly begin to straighten your arms. When you get to the top part of the motion, your arms should be extended directly over your chest, and your hands, palms facing each other, should almost be touching. Hold for a beat, and lower the weight to the starting position as you inhale. Come to a dead stop at the bottom of the motion to prevent your arms from bouncing off the ball.

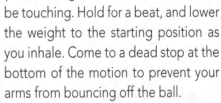

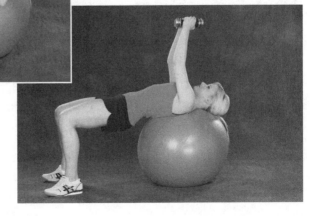

Hollywood Incline Fly

This has a similar motion to the Hollywood Fly, but with one difference. Thanks to the slightly different angle, you'll be targeting more of the middle and upper parts of the chest.

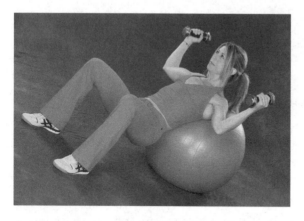

GET READY

From a sitting position on a stability ball, with a dumbbell in each hand, roll down until your upper back is resting on the ball and your upper body is at a 45-degree angle to the floor. Place the tip of your tongue behind your top front teeth. Your feet should be shoulder-width apart and flat on the floor. Extend your arms out to the side, with the palms facing up and the elbows bent and pointed down.

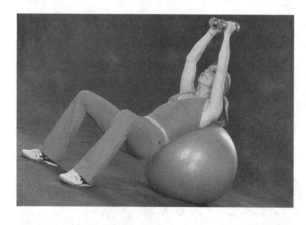

DO THE EXERCISE

Take a deep breath. Exhale and drive the weight straight up as if you were hugging a stability ball. At around the halfway point, slowly begin to straighten your arms. When you get to the top part of the motion, your arms should be extended above you as if reaching for the ceiling, and your hands, palms facing each other, should almost be touching. Hold for a beat, and lower the weight to the starting position as you inhale. Come to a dead stop at the bottom of the motion to prevent your arms from bouncing off the ball.

Hollywood C Sweep

This is the ultimate exercise for sculpting the pectorals. Picture each hand tracing a semicircle (or the letter C), and you should have no trouble with this one.

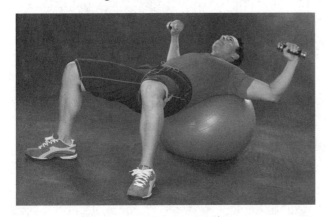

GET READY

Lie back on a stability ball with a dumbbell in each hand. The ball should be under your upper back and supporting your head in a natural position. Your feet should be shoulder-width apart and your hips should be raised. With your elbows bent and pointed toward the ground, bring your hands slightly higher than your shoulders so that the dumbbells are even with your ears, your palms are facing out, and your knuckles are facing the ceiling.

DO THE EXERCISE

Take a deep breath. Exhale and use your chest muscles to slowly trace an arcing pattern, moving the dumbbells from ear level to waist level. Do not lower or raise the dumbbells; keep them the same distance off the floor until the very end of the motion. At the bottom of the C, raise your hands slightly, the palms facing toward your head, and feel the squeeze in the lower part of your pecs. Inhale and slowly reverse the motion.

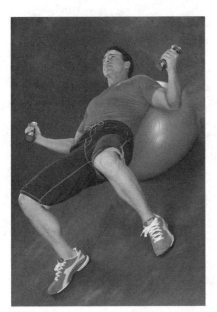

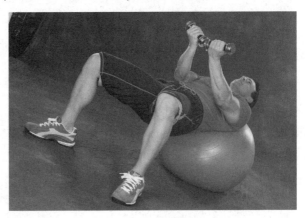

Celebrity Back

When it comes to high-profile celebrity backs, think Hillary Swank or Daniel Craig. Just as with the chest, you'll notice that what makes a back so spectacular is different for men and women. In both cases, though, developing the muscles of the back helps you to move closer toward that celebrity body in not one, not even two, but three significant ways.

First off, building and toning the muscles that make up the middle and upper back will give you a more athletic and tapered look. For women, the goal isn't about size or thickening these muscles. It's about working the muscles of the upper back to create clear lines of definition. These are slenderizing lines that will give you a strong, yet sexy look in a bathing suit or a backless dress. For men, it's about size and thickening and also sculpting. The back is a huge canvas on which to work. The goal is to achieve thickness in the middle and upper back and sculpted definition along the sides, from the armpits down to the midpoint of your rib cage. From all angles it will give you a tapered, V-shaped look. And if you happen to be carrying some extra weight around your waist, building up and sculpting the muscles that run down the sides of your body will make your midsection appear thinner.

Second, strengthening the muscles of the mid and upper back will improve your posture by drawing your shoulder girdle back and helping you to stand taller. Standing taller, even if you don't lose a single pound, will automatically make you appear slimmer. Strengthening the muscles of the lower back is a must for keeping you healthy and pain-free. Lower-back pain is an interesting thing. Most chronic sufferers will hurt their back, rest it for a while, hurt it again, rest it, and so on. This cycle goes on forever, or until the back finally gives out completely. The best way to break this cycle is to strengthen the muscles in your lower back. When they're strong enough to do everything you need them to do, you won't hurt your lower back when bending over to pick up the newspaper or leaning forward to get something out of the fridge.

Finally, adding lean muscle will increase your metabolism and force you to burn more calories, and the large area that makes up your back is a great place to do it. For every pound of lean muscle you put on—and, again, we're not talking bulky muscle—your body will burn between 35 and 50 extra calories per day, every day. In addition, every time you work the muscles in your back, which you'll be doing three times per week, your body has to burn even more calories over the next twenty-four to forty-eight hours as it works to repair the muscle fiber you tore down while working out.

Back Muscles

The trapezius, or "traps," are the muscles that form a triangular shape on either side of your upper back, the three points of the triangle being the center of the back, the shoulders, and the neck. Their main job is to move and stabilize the shoulder blades. Well-developed traps will add definition to the upper back, but they are most visible at their uppermost part, where they appear as the muscle that runs from the top of the shoulders to the neck. If you want to feel your traps in action, simply shrug your shoulders. We'll be doing just that, with weights, when we do the Hollywood Shrug.

The latissimus dorsi are the winglike muscles that flank the back. The job of your lats is to bring your arms down and in toward your body. To see what they feel like, stand with your arms out in a T position, then drop them to your sides. Did you feel anything in your back? Probably not. Now I want you to do the same thing, but as you bring your arms down to your sides, pretend that you're going against a resisting force that wants you to keep them up. What you feel now are your lats. Because of the job they do, they're involved in just about any pulling motion you make. And since they're generally considered to be the marquee muscles of the back, we'll be working them out in several different ways, from the Hollywood One-Armed Row and Hollywood Bent-Over Row to the Hollywood Pull-Over.

The erector spinae consists of three muscles—the iliocostalis, the longissimus, and the spinalis—that run alongside the back of your spine. They have the daunting job of keeping you standing upright. Most lower-back problems are a result of these muscles not being strong enough to do what you need them to do. We'll be working the erectors a lot. They're the main target of the Hollywood Hyperextensions, but any exercise where you lean forward and have to stabilize your body—the Hollywood Bent-Over Row, for example—works to strengthen this very important group of muscles.

Hollywood One-Armed Row

Working one arm at a time will really let you focus on the differences in strength between your right and left sides. Over time, this will erase any strength or size variations and will leave you balanced, both in power and aesthetically. Concentrate on moving the weight with the large muscles of your back, not with your smaller biceps muscles. This is a back exercise. We'll hit your biceps later.

GET READY
With a dumbbell in your right hand, lean forward and place your left hand on a stability ball. Your back should be straight and almost parallel to the ground. Your legs should be bent slightly, with your feet shoulder-width apart. The right hand should be hanging directly under your shoulder, with your palm facing in.

DO THE EXERCISE
Take a deep breath. Exhale and slowly draw the weight up by squeezing your shoulder blade and raising your bent elbow toward the ceiling. Imagine that you're sawing a piece of wood. Hold this "up" position for a beat, then lower the weight to the starting position as you inhale. Try to keep your shoulders parallel to the ground throughout the entire exercise. Row for 30 seconds with your right arm, then row for 30 seconds with your left arm.

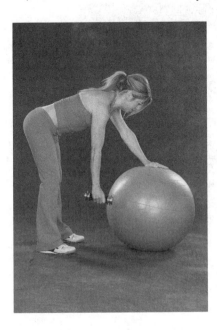 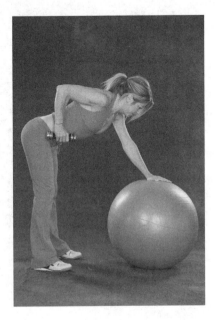

Hollywood Bent-Over Row

Similar to the One-Armed Row, but since you don't have a spare arm to stabilize yourself, it's up to your lower back to do the stabilization. Focus on keeping your mid and upper back strong and straight to keep your lower back happy. And, again, concentrate on raising the weight by squeezing your shoulder blades, not by trying to pull it up with your arm.

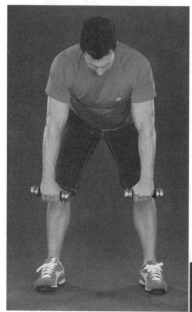

GET READY

With a dumbbell in each hand and your palms facing in toward your thighs, bend your knees and lean forward until your upper body is at a roughly 45-degree angle. The dumbbells should be hanging directly under your shoulders.

DO THE EXERCISE

Take a deep breath. Exhale and slowly draw the weights up by squeezing your shoulder blades together and raising your bent elbows toward the ceiling. Keep your shoulders parallel to the floor and your back straight. Hold for a beat at the top of the motion, then slowly lower the weights back to the starting position as you inhale.

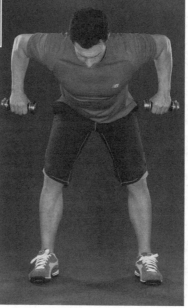

Hollywood Pull-Over

This is a great exercise that manages to strengthen, stretch, and stabilize the upper body all at the same time. You'll definitely feel it working your lats, but it's one of the best exercises for stretching the chest muscles and building the stabilizers in the shoulders.

GET READY

Holding a single dumbbell with both hands, lie back on a stability ball. The ball should be resting under your upper back so that your head is in a natural position. Press the weight up toward the ceiling. Your arms should be straight, but your elbows should not be locked out.

DO THE EXERCISE

Inhale and slowly lower the weight above your head and toward the floor. When your arms are parallel to the floor, hold for a beat and feel a great stretch in your chest, then slowly return to the starting position as you exhale.

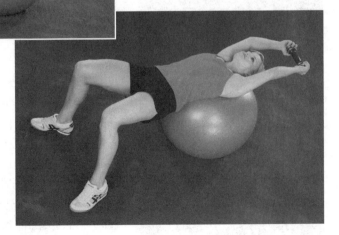

Hollywood Shrug

One of the true secrets to the Hollywood body is working the trapezius muscles, which run from the shoulders to the neck. For men, this muscle ties together the

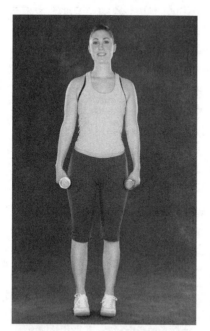

back and the shoulders and makes them look that much more impressive. For women, it makes the neck look longer and adds some very sexy muscular definition around the shoulder blades: the perfect complement to a backless dress or a swimsuit. For both sexes, though, this shrug will not only strengthen the traps, it will also stretch them. And since the upper back and the neck are where so many of us carry stress, this just might be the most therapeutic exercise in the whole book!

GET READY

Stand with your knees slightly bent, feet shoulder-width apart, and a dumbbell in each hand by your side, palms facing toward your thighs.

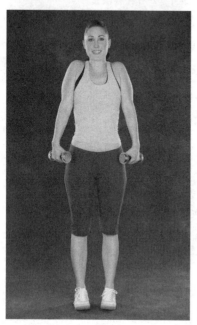

DO THE EXERCISE

Take a deep breath. Exhale and slowly lift your shoulders toward your ears as high as possible. Imagine that someone just asked you what the highest mountain in Spain is or who was the first vice president under McKinley. What would you do? You'd shrug your shoulders. Hold for a beat and then lower the weight, feeling a stretch through your shoulders and neck as you inhale. (And just in case anyone ever *does* ask, the highest mountain in Spain is El Teide in Tenerife, and Garret Hobart was the first vice president under McKinley.)

Hollywood Hyperextension

I'll be the first to admit that a Hollywood Hyperextension sounds like something you wouldn't wish on your worst enemy, but this may be the best exercise you can do for your lower back. Keeping your lower back healthy and strong is not only a key to achieving the Hollywood body, it's essential to having a happy life. If you've ever suffered from lower-back pain, you know how debilitating it can be. This exercise will help you to stay pain-free.

This is also the only exercise that you'll do with a reverse breathing pattern. You'll be inhaling as you lift your body. The reason is that if you inhale on the negative phase, as you lower your body around the ball, you'll put too much pressure on your stomach.

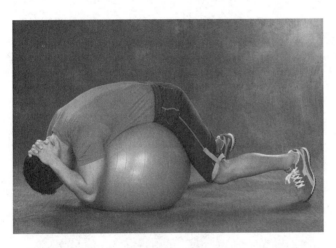

GET READY

Drape yourself over a stability ball so that it rests directly under your stomach. Come up on your toes and bring your knees off the floor. Clasp your hands behind your head, being careful not to put too much pressure on your neck, and slowly drop your head toward the floor. Feel your spine lengthening as it curls around the ball. You may want to hold this position for a few seconds and enjoy the stretch.

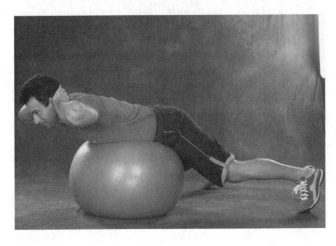

DO THE EXERCISE

Inhale and slowly uncurl your spine by straightening your back and lifting your upper body. When your upper body is parallel to the floor, hold for a beat, then return to the starting position as you exhale.

Celebrity Shoulders

Although not as large as the muscles of the chest and the back, the shoulder muscles do their part aesthetically and functionally in helping you to achieve the celebrity look. And for both good looks and a healthier and stronger you, we're going to focus especially on the back part of the shoulders. They're the muscles that are probably the most neglected in strength-training programs.

Here's a test: stand with your arms out to your sides and your palms facing the floor, as if you were a giant letter T. Now drop your arms to your sides. If you're like most people, your palms ended up near your front pockets. This means that your shoulders roll in slightly and that you're stronger in the front of your body. The reason we're going to spend so much time on the rear part of the shoulder is to fix this slight imbalance. By strengthening the back part of the shoulder muscles, we'll draw your shoulder girdle back, letting you stand up taller and be more balanced in the front-versus-back strength department. By the end of my program, when you perform the same drop-your-arms test, your palms will end up a lot closer to the sides of your thighs than to the fronts.

Aesthetically, strong shoulders will give you a more commanding presence. They form the summit of the V-shaped physique that looks so impressive on both men and women. Look at Mark Wahlberg, for example, and the way his shoulders almost magically make his back look more developed and his waist slimmer. And does anyone have a more commanding presence than Madonna? Her shoulders are powerful, sculpted, and sexy. Are they the size of bowling balls? No. For women, the look isn't about size. It's about tone and definition.

The shoulders also contain the hidden jewel of the upper body. Forget about the biceps, the real star of the show is the rear part of the shoulders. The arms come from the shoulders. By developing the back of the shoulder, you create a defined ridge where it meets the back of the arm. Whether you're male or female, this sexy definition between the shoulders and the arms will draw eyes to it like a magnet.

Developing the muscles in the back of the shoulder isn't just about looks, though. On the functional side, strong shoulders that are developed in a balanced way will help to improve your posture. By working the back of the muscle group, you will draw your shoulder blades back and almost immediately stand taller and with better posture—and standing taller will instantly make you appear leaner and thinner.

Shoulder Muscles

Deltoid muscles are broken up into three parts: the anterior (front), the lateral (side), and the posterior (rear). Each part has its own function. The front part of the deltoid is what allows you to raise your arm up straight in front of you. Put your arms up in front of you as if you're sleepwalking or you're a zombie. If you reach across with one hand and touch the front of your opposite shoulder, you'll feel how hard it is. Raising your arms out to the side, as you did in the standing test for front-versus-back strength, is the job of the side delts. The rear delts work with the muscles of the back to counterbalance the strength of the chest. Remember how one of the functions of the chest was to move your arms from that standing T position to a position where they were extended directly in front of you? The job of the rear delts is to do the opposite. If you start with your arms extended in front of you, like a zombie, and then extend them out to your sides to the T position, you've just worked your rear delts.

Rotator cuff muscles are a group of four muscles whose job it is to rotate the arm at the shoulder. Place your arm straight out in front of you with your palm facing down. (If you were paying attention, you'll remember that it's the front part of the deltoid that's letting you hold your arm out that way.) Keeping your arm straight, turn your palm up toward the ceiling. Now turn it back to facing the floor. You've just used your rotators. Compared to the large muscles in the area—the pecs, the lats, and the deltoids—the muscles that make up your rotator cuff are like rubber bands. They can very easily be injured if you don't keep them strong. That's the job of my Hollywood Field Goals. No one will ever stop you on the street and compliment you on your sexy rotators—they're virtually invisible—but if you want to have a celebrity body, you need to keep them healthy and happy.

Hollywood W Shoulders

This is the exercise I developed years ago in Boston, and I still haven't found a better way to work all three parts of the shoulder: the anterior deltoid, the lateral deltoid, and the posterior deltoid.

GET READY

Stand with a dumbbell in each hand, with your elbows pointing down and your hands, palms facing in, at shoulder level. Your arms should make a W shape.

DO THE EXERCISE

Take a deep breath. Exhale and drive the weight straight up toward the ceiling, but no higher than head height. At the top of the motion, your upper arms should be parallel to the floor and your hands, palms still facing in, should be slightly wider than your elbows. Hold for a beat, then slowly reverse the motion and return to the starting position as you inhale.

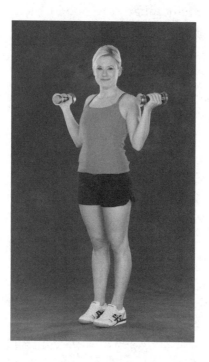 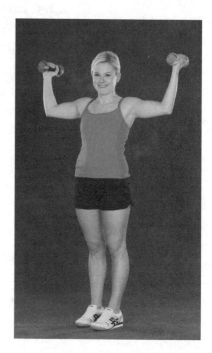

Hollywood Field Goals

If your favorite baseball pitcher ever spent a year on the disabled list because of a rotator cuff injury, you can be pretty sure it's because he wasn't doing exercises like this. The Field Goal strengthens the small muscles that rotate the shoulder. That will keep you injury-free not only while you do the rest of the exercises in the book, but also while you walk the dog or toss a ball around with your kids.

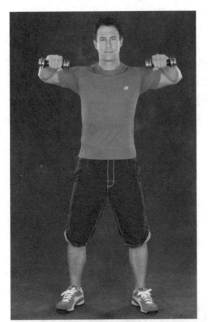

GET READY

Stand with your feet shoulder-width apart and your knees slightly bent. With a dumbbell in each hand, raise your arms so that your upper arms are extended out from your sides and parallel to the floor. Bend your elbows 90 degrees so that your forearms are pointing forward and are parallel to the floor. Your palms should be facing the floor. Basically, you should look as if you're about to push the world's largest shopping cart.

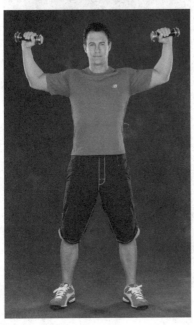

DO THE EXERCISE

Take a deep breath. Exhale and, keeping your upper arms from moving, rotate at the elbows so that your forearms are now pointing straight up at the ceiling. Your palms should now be facing forward. You'll feel some sensation in the rear part of your shoulders. That's your body's way of saying, "Thanks for thinking of my smaller muscles!" Reverse the motion and return to the starting position on the inhalation.

Hollywood Funky Chicken

It's just like the wedding dance but with weights. This exercise works on the outer part of the shoulder muscle to help you attain that athletic and sexy tapering V-shaped upper body.

GET READY

Stand with your feet shoulder-width apart and your knees slightly bent. Have a dumbbell in each hand. Your upper arms should be perpendicular to the floor and alongside your ribs. Your elbows should be bent at 90-degree angles so that your forearms point forward and are parallel to the floor. Your palms should be facing in.

DO THE EXERCISE

Take a deep breath. Exhale and, keeping the 90-degree bend in your elbows, raise your upper arms to the sides until they are parallel to the floor. Hold this position for a beat, then slowly lower the weights back to the starting position as you inhale.

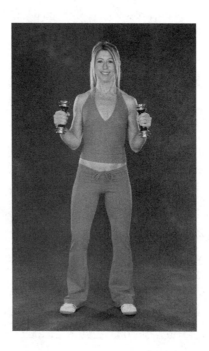 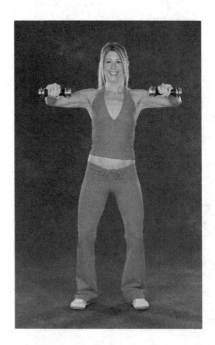

Hollywood Bent-Over Rear Delt

One of the best ways to improve your posture and realign the shoulders is by working the muscles in the rear part of the shoulders. This exercise is a great way to do just that.

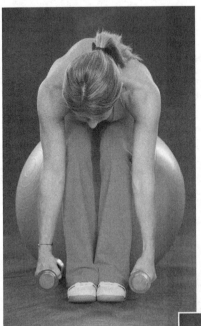

GET READY

Sit on a stability ball with a dumbbell in each hand and lean forward. Try to bring your chest right down to your thighs, but if you can't go quite that far, don't worry. Let your arms dangle straight down from your shoulders with your palms facing each other.

DO THE EXERCISE

Take a deep breath. Exhale and slowly raise your arms out to the sides, keeping them straight, until they're parallel to the ground and your palms are facing the floor. At the top of the motion, squeeze your shoulder blades together. Hold this position for a beat, then reverse the motion and return to the starting position as you inhale.

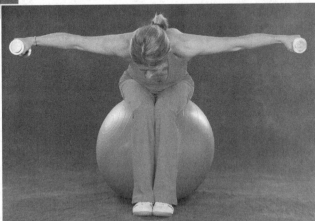

Celebrity Arms

Since we live in a world that generally requires us to wear shirts, pants, dresses, and so on, most parts of our bodies are covered with clothes a lot of the time. That's not true of our arms. In the summer up North or year-round in the South, our arms are naked for everyone to see, so it's important that they look their best. Fortunately, the muscles of the arms are some of the easiest to develop.

The key to sexy arms, whether you're male or female, is balance. You need to have the proper balance between the muscles in the front of the arm and those in the back of the arm. When it works, it's like a perfect relationship. Two of the nicest pairs of arms in Hollywood belong to Brad Pitt and Jessica Biel. For both women and men, arms are about tone and definition.

For women, balanced weight training, along with the other fat-burning techniques we use, will take care of the flabbiness that can show up on the back side of the arm and will give the entire arm a lean, defined, muscular look.

For men, the goal is no longer pure size. The idea is to have size but have it be proportional to the rest of your body. Mutantlike arms may be okay if you're a bouncer, but for the lean, cut celebrity look, you want sculpted definition. My plan chisels away at the most visible part of the arm muscles: the outer sides. These are the parts of the muscle the world sees most often. When you add definition here to the definition we've already created around the front side and the rear parts of the shoulder muscles, you get simply jaw-dropping results.

Arm Muscles

The biceps are the muscles on the front of your upper arm that run from the base of your shoulder muscles to your elbow (exactly how close to the elbow differs from person to person and is determined by genetics). The job of the biceps is to flex the arm at the elbow. Any time you go from a straight-arm position to a bent-at-the-elbow position, you're using your biceps. This happens in complex motions, like the Hollywood Bent-Over Row, that we use for strengthening the back. It also happens in simpler motions, like the Hollywood Hammer Curl, that are designed primarily to work the biceps. You'll notice while doing your workouts that we generally do the more complex motions involving the biceps before doing the ones that are designed to isolate the muscle. This isn't by accident. You need your biceps to be fresh when working the large muscles of your back. You don't want them doing the work of your back muscles, but you need them there to help. When their job is done, you can concentrate on working the biceps by themselves. This gets the most out of them.

The triceps are the muscles on the back of the upper arm that run from just under the shoulder muscle down to the elbow. Their job is the opposite of the biceps'—that is, they take you from a bent-at-the-elbow position to a straight-arm position. And for the same reasons that we do complex back motions before doing exercises that target the biceps exclusively, we do our complex pushing motions— Push-Ups, Hollywood W Shoulders—first before concentrating on exercises like the Hollywood Kickbacks with a Twist that isolate the triceps. It's that twist that makes this exercise so great. The twisting motion that you do at the top of the motion is what targets the outer head of the triceps and really helps to sculpt the outside part of the upper arm.

Biceps Curl with a Hollywood Twist

We're going to take a traditional exercise and add some extra value. The twist that you do with your wrist at the very top of this motion will ensure that you get the absolute most out of your biceps. Look down at your biceps when you do the twist, and you may see the muscle contract a bit more.

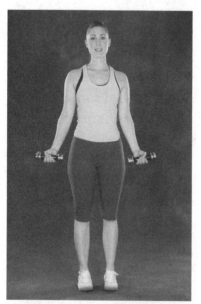

GET READY

From a standing position, with your feet hip-width apart and your arms down by your sides, hold a dumbbell in each hand, palms facing forward.

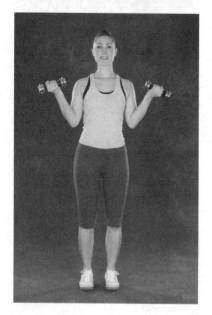

DO THE EXERCISE

Take a deep breath. Exhale and slowly raise the weights by bending your arms at the elbows. The key to getting the most out of your biceps is to keep the upper arms from moving. When the weights are at shoulder height, twist your wrists inward, as if you wanted to have the backs of your hands face each other. You won't be able to twist very far in this direction; you're not supposed to be able to. All you're looking for is a little extra squeeze for your biceps. Hold for a beat, then slowly lower the weight—keeping your upper arms from moving—back to the starting position as you inhale.

Hollywood Hammer Curl

This is another slight tweak on a traditional biceps curl. The difference here is the way you hold the dumbbells. Instead of starting with your palms facing forward and then turning them to face you at the top of the motion, here your palms will face in toward you for the entire movement. It may not seem like a big difference, but you'll quickly feel the difference, especially in your forearms.

GET READY

From a standing position, with your feet hip-width apart and your arms down by your sides, hold a dumbbell in each hand, palms facing in toward your thighs.

DO THE EXERCISE

Take a deep breath. Exhale and slowly raise the weights by bending your arms at the elbows. As with all curls, make sure that your upper arms don't move. All the motion should come from the elbows down. When the dumbbells are at shoulder height—your palms should be facing each other—hold for a beat, then reverse the motion and slowly return to the starting position as you inhale.

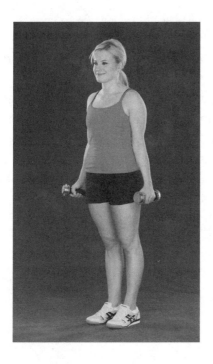 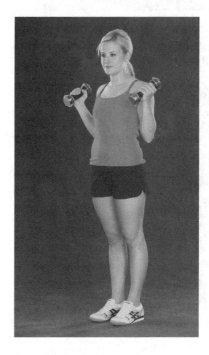

Hollywood Upside-Down Curl

Another curl—another variation. This is a great way to strengthen the muscles in your forearms as you work your biceps.

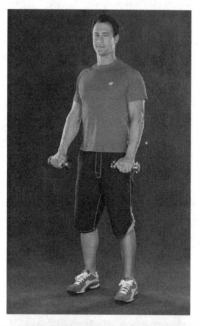

GET READY

From a standing position with your feet hip-width apart and your arms down by your sides, hold a dumbbell in each hand, palms facing behind you.

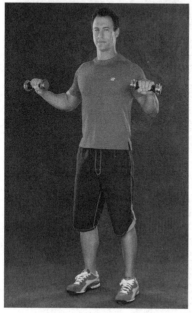

DO THE EXERCISE

Take a deep breath. Exhale and slowly raise the weights by bending your arms at the elbows. Your upper arms may move slightly during this curl. It's the mechanics of the motion. Try to minimize any movement of the upper arms. When the weights are at shoulder height and your palms are facing away from you, hold for a beat, then slowly reverse the motion and return to the starting position as you inhale.

Hollywood Karate Curl

This is a little bit different from your average curl, but the rules are the same: try to minimize the movement of your upper arms. This will force your biceps to do all the work and will not let the muscles in your shoulders help them out.

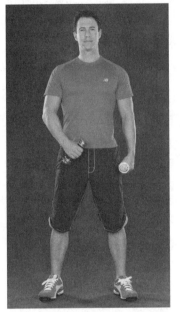

GET READY

From a standing position, with your feet hip-width apart and a dumbbell in each hand, turn your right wrist so that your palm is facing you at waist level.

DO THE EXERCISE

Take a deep breath. Exhale and, while starting with the weight in your right hand in front of your stomach and chest and your palm facing in, sweep the weight in an arcing motion until it's at shoulder height. Hold for a beat and instead of reversing the motion to lower the weight, lower it by slowly letting your forearm drop forward as you inhale. Repeat with your left arm.

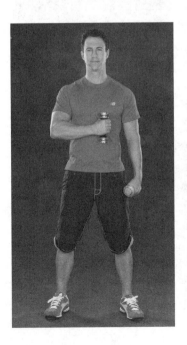
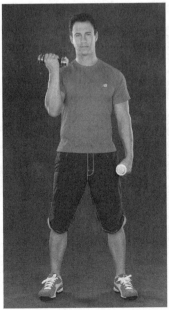
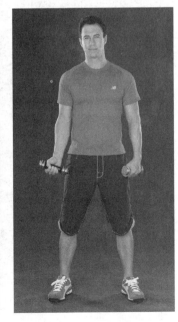

Hollywood Kickback with a Twist

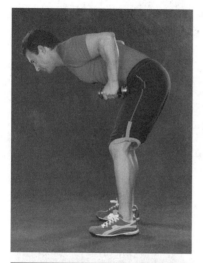

The Kickback is one of the best exercises for working the triceps, and by adding a couple of wrist twists at the end, I've made it even better. On your own, try a few without the twists and then a few with the twists to see how much harder the triceps have to work in the twisting version.

GET READY

With a dumbbell in each hand and your feet slightly wider than shoulder-width apart, bend your knees slightly and bend over at the hip, keeping your back as straight as possible, until your upper body is parallel to the floor. Raise your elbows until they are against your sides and your upper arms are also parallel to the floor. Bend your elbows 90 degrees so that your hands are directly below your elbows and your palms are facing in toward you.

DO THE EXERCISE

Take a deep breath. Exhale and raise the weights in back of you by straightening your arms. The key is to keep your upper arms in place and not to move them. All the motion should come from the elbows down. When your arms are

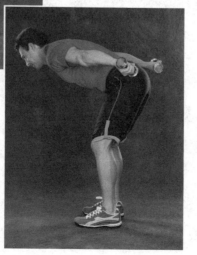

straight and parallel to the floor, twist your wrists so that your palms are now facing the floor. Hold for a beat and twist your wrists in the opposite direction so that your palms face the ceiling. Hold for a beat, then slowly return to the starting position as you inhale, making that sure that your upper arms stay in place. Come to a complete dead stop at the down position before doing your next repetition.

Hollywood Ball Press

In addition to strengthening the triceps, this nifty move will also strengthen your abs, lower back, and shoulders.

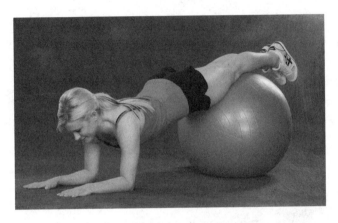

GET READY

Drape yourself over a stability ball and walk yourself forward until the ball is under your upper thigh. Keeping your body straight, slowly lower yourself by bending at the elbows until your forearms are on the ground, shoulder-width apart and parallel to your body.

Where you are in relation to the ball will affect the difficulty of the exercise. If you're finding it too difficult to do the motion with the ball under your upper thigh, scoot back until the ball is closer to your waist. As you get stronger, slide forward so that the ball is under your thighs, knees, or shins.

DO THE EXERCISE

Take a deep breath. Exhale and push off the floor until your arms are straight and your hands are directly beneath your shoulders. Slowly lower yourself to the starting position as you inhale.

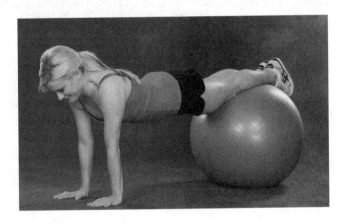

Alternating Hollywood Triceps Raise

This is a great way to work your triceps, and having to balance on the ball will work your legs and core.

GET READY

With a dumbbell in each hand, lie back on a stability ball so that the ball is under your lower back and your head is resting in a neutral and comfortable position. Raise your hips so that there's a straight line running from your knees to your shoulders. That line should be parallel to the floor. Straighten your arms and press the weights toward the ceiling. Your arms should be fully extended and perpendicular to the floor, with your palms facing each other.

DO THE EXERCISE

Take a deep breath. Exhale and slowly lower the weight in your right hand by bending at the elbow. Try to keep your elbow pointed at the ceiling and your upper arms parallel to each other. When your right forearm is parallel to the floor, hold for a beat, then return to the starting position as you inhale. Repeat with your left arm.

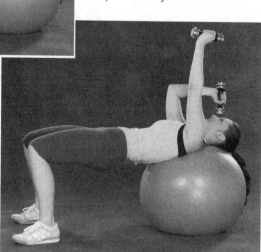

Hollywood Overhead Tri

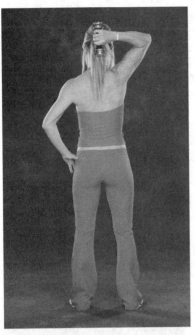

Go slowly on this one to avoid straining your neck, and be careful not to hit yourself on the head with the dumbbell.

GET READY

With a dumbbell in your right hand, stand with your feet shoulder-width apart. Bring the weight up and behind your head. Your palm should be facing the back of your head, and your wrist should be turned so that your thumb faces the floor and your pinkie faces the ceiling. From the front, it might look as if you were trying to hide something behind your head.

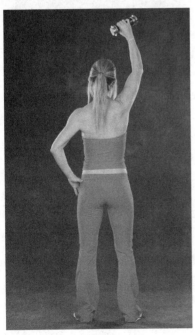

DO THE EXERCISE

Take a deep breath. Exhale and drive the weight up by beginning to straighten your right arm. You don't want to fully lock out your arm. If straight up is twelve o'clock, you want your hand to stop at eleven o'clock. Hold for a beat, then reverse the motion and return to the starting position as you inhale. Do 30 seconds with your right arm, then 30 seconds with your left arm.

Celebrity Lower Body

Since the majority of the lower-body exercises target and strengthen more than one specific body part, I thought they would be easier to understand if I explained my strategy and the science behind lower-body training as a whole, before I introduced you to the exercises. So let's start at the top.

Celebrity Butt

Whether you're a man or a woman, you want a shapely and attractive behind. If your chest is the first thing a potential mate looks at when he or she sees you from the front, your butt is the first thing that is seen when the person looks at you from behind.

For both men and women, the key is to create a dividing line—a clear line of separation—between the buttocks and the back of your legs. Developing the muscles this way will lift your rear, giving you a more youthful look. For women, who genetically carry a little more natural fat in this area, it will also accentuate your behind, making it appear firmer and fuller. The goal is a "tear drop" shape. The actress Jessica Biel has this shape. Men want to work the outside of the buttocks to create that indent at the very top of the side of the thigh. I've been told by reliable sources that if you were looking for a celebrity role model to pattern your butt after, your list should start and end with Orlando Bloom.

Butt Muscles

The gluteus maximus is generally the muscle that people think of when they talk about the buttocks, although you'll soon see that it's not the only factor in having a shapely behind. Glutes have two jobs. The first is to straighten the body at the hips. Any time you go from a bent-at-the-hips position, like sitting, to a straight-body position, like standing, you're working the glutes. The muscle's other job is to rotate the leg outward. To get a feel for that, stand with your toes facing forward and then angle them out slightly. Again, you're working the glutes. My program has no shortage of ways to work the glutes. Squats, lunges, and the Hollywood Arrow all take you from a bent-at-the-hips to a straight-body position, and all are designed to strengthen, shape, and lift the buttocks.

The gluteus medius are the muscles on either side of your glutes, and it's essential to work them as well, to have a defined and sculpted behind. The job of the gluteus medius is to stabilize the hips and raise the legs out to the side. Unfortunately, people don't do a whole lot of lifting their legs sideways. They move them forward and back when they walk or run, but rarely out to the side. That's what's so great about the Hollywood Side Raises you'll be doing. I'm sure that the first time you do them, it'll be as if you're discovering a brand-new body part.

Celebrity Thighs

For most of us, even people you'd consider to be in good shape, the legs can be an underdeveloped work in progress. Since we can hide this weakness under pants, long skirts, and so on, many of us never get around to developing our legs correctly. When it comes to strengthening the legs, for both men and women the goal is balance. Men might strive for more size, but the real key is balance between the muscles in the front of the thigh and those in the back. Look at Cameron Diaz, for example, or Jake Gyllenhaal.

The motions of daily life—walking, running—tend to target the muscles in the front of the thigh. That's why even if you've never strength trained before, the fronts of your thighs will look more developed than the backs of your thighs. We need to develop both sides to create a sexy and proportional look. The muscles in the front of the thigh should bow out slightly from just below the hip bone to just above the knee. The muscles in the back of your thigh should also bow out, from just under the buttocks to just above the knee. When a perfect balance is hit, you'll see a dividing line—a sexy dividing line—appear along the side of your thigh, dividing the muscles in the front from those in the back.

While building your legs will undoubtedly give you a sexier and more proportional look, it'll do double duty by letting you greatly increase the number of calories you'll burn throughout the day. The muscle groups of the legs are the largest muscle groups on your body, and just like the muscles of the back, they're great potential storehouses for calorie-hungry lean muscle. Since most of us have underdeveloped legs, simply by building stronger, shapelier legs—something we want to do anyway—we'll be turbo-charging our metabolisms at the same time.

Thigh Muscles

Hip adductors, on the inside of the thigh, are the muscles that work in opposition to the gluteus medius. Hip adductors are a group of several muscles whose job it is to draw the leg back toward the body. Strengthening these muscles, as you'll do with the Hollywood Squeeze Play, can help to reduce unflattering flabby inner thighs.

The tensor fascia latae are the muscles on the front of the hip that flex the hip forward. Although the look of these muscles doesn't greatly affect the way you appear, how strong and how tight they are definitely does. Tight hip flexors cause you to walk with a slight forward lean. In addition to not exactly being the sexiest way to strut around, over time it can lead to lower-back problems. Most of the crunches and crunch variations that you'll do will also work the hip flexors as they work the muscles in your abdomen. More important, though, are the things you'll do to stretch your hip flexors. All of the lunges that you'll do, in addition to the Hollywood Butt Kicks, will help to make your hip flexors loose and keep you standing and walking tall.

The quadriceps are the four muscles that make up the front part of the thigh. They're very visible because they're on the front of your body. Developed quads will give you a healthy athletic look and an overall balanced look to your body. Underdeveloped quads can make you look scrawny. This is especially a problem for men. Scrawny legs detract from an otherwise impressive physique. The quads are involved in flexing your hips, but their primary job is to extend or straighten the leg at the knee. Going from a bent-knee position to a straight-knee position works the quads. That's what is so great about motions like lunges and squats; in addition to working the glutes, they also give the quads a good workout.

The hamstrings are the three muscles that make up the back of the thigh. Like a lot of the muscles on the back side of our body, the hamstrings can get neglected when it comes to training. Underdeveloped hamstrings can not only give an unbalanced look to the leg, but can greatly detract from a strong and shapely behind. The job of the hamstrings is to work with the glutes to straighten the body, as you'll do in the Hollywood Arrow, and to bend the leg at the knee, which you'll do in the Hollywood Hamstring Curl.

Celebrity Calves

Just like the muscles in the back of the thigh, the calf muscles have a tendency to be underdeveloped. Surprisingly, among people who've never worked out before, women generally have more developed calves than men. They can thank the makers of high-heeled shoes for that. Walking around all day with your toes several inches below your heels will work the calves without your ever having to step one of your high-heeled feet into the weight room. For the rest of us, though, strengthening and developing the calves are crucial to finishing off the look of the leg. For women, well-proportioned calves will draw the eye away from heavier thighs and will give a slimmer appearance to thick ankles. For men, strong calves are a sign of virility. And even if your upper thighs are yet to develop or are still a work in progress, nice-size calves worn with baggy to-the-knee shorts can give you the appearance of having powerful and sexy legs.

Calf Muscles

The job of the calf muscles, gastrocnemius/soleus, is to extend the foot or point the toes downward. You have two muscles that help to do this. The soleus is the deeper of the two muscles, and it runs from just below the knee to the top of the heel. On top of this is the gastrocnemius, the more superficial—or closer to the surface—muscle. It runs from just behind the knee to about mid-calf. Any time you go up on tip-toes, you're working the muscles in your calves. As far as strength training goes, we'll hit the muscles of the calf when we do the Hollywood Sumo Squat with Calf Raise. We'll also target these muscles in a lot of the cardio we do. The jogging will really hit them, but they'll also be called into play in the stepping and lunging phases of the program.

Hollywood "I Dream of Jeannie" Squat

This is a great way to work the glutes (your butt), as well as the quadriceps (the large muscles that make up the fronts of your thighs). The key when squatting is to make sure your knees stay over your heels or over the middle of each foot. If your knees slide over your toes or farther, it can put a lot of pressure on your knees. Focus on having very good technique.

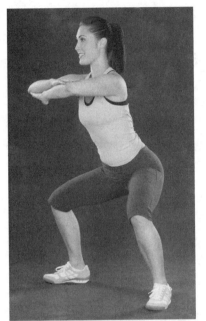

GET READY

Stand with your feet slightly wider than shoulder-width apart, with knees unlocked, toes angled out at 45-degree angles, and your arms crossed in front of your chest—just like Jeannie. Make sure you keep your head up and your eyes looking forward to avoid throwing your balance off.

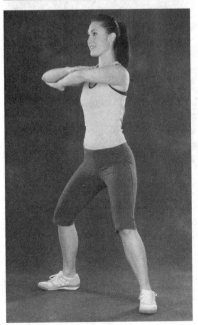

DO THE EXERCISE

Inhale and kick your hips back. Then slowly lower your butt as if you were about to sit in an imaginary chair behind you. Remember, you want to keep your knees centered over your heels as much as possible. When your thighs are parallel to the floor—don't worry if you can't get that deep, just do your best—hold for a beat, then return to the starting position by driving off your heels and straightening your legs as you exhale.

Hollywood Sumo Squat with Calf Raise

The wider stance of this squat will really make you aware of your inner thighs. The calf raise at the end may initially test your balance, but once you get the hang of it, it's a great tool for building your calves.

GET READY

Stand with your feet almost twice shoulder-width apart, toes angled out at 45 degrees and your arms crossed in front of your chest. Make sure you keep your head up and your eyes looking forward to avoid throwing your balance off.

DO THE EXERCISE

Inhale and kick your hips back. Then, slowly lower your butt, as if you were about to sit in an imaginary chair behind you. Just as with the "I Dream of Jeannie" Squat, you want to keep your knees centered over your heels as much as possible. When your thighs are parallel to the floor, hold for a beat, then drive off your heels as you raise your butt. With your knees still bent at a 45-degree angle, push up onto the balls of your feet, lifting your heels off the ground as you exhale. Hold this position for a beat, then repeat.

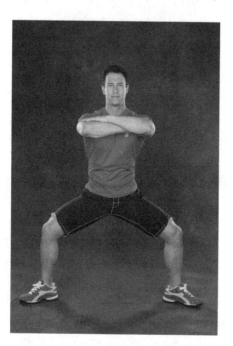
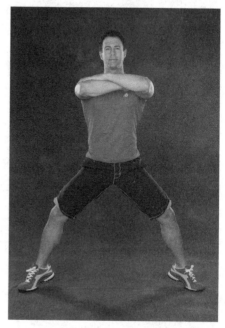

Hollywood Butt Kick

This great exercise is a simple and effective way to strengthen and tone the butt.

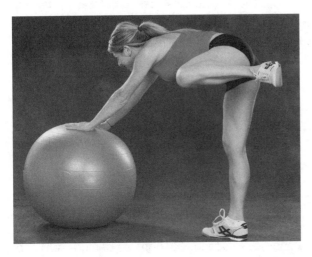

GET READY

With your feet shoulder-width apart, lean forward at the hip and place both hands on a stability ball for balance. Draw your left leg up and in toward your chest. Rotate your lower leg so that it's parallel to your upper body. Bend your foot at a 90-degree angle.

DO THE EXERCISE

Take a deep breath. Exhale and straighten your leg out behind you, as if you wanted to leave a footprint on the wall. When your leg is fully extended, there should be a straight line running from your heel to the top of your head. Inhale and reverse the motion to return to the starting position. Kick for 30 seconds with your left leg, then 30 seconds with your right leg.

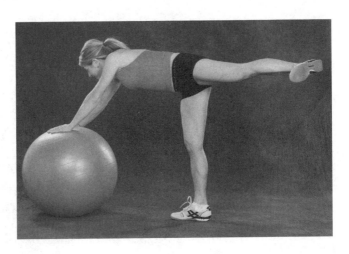

Hollywood Arrow

This is not only a great way to stretch and strengthen your glutes and hamstrings (the muscles that make up the backs of your thighs), it's a great way to develop balance and body awareness. If you have trouble doing this at first, you can hold onto the back of a chair with your free hand until your technique improves.

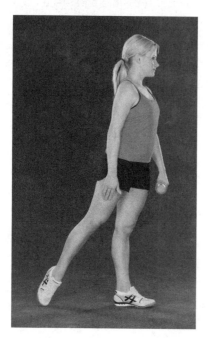

GET READY
Stand with a dumbbell in your left hand and your feet closer than hip-width apart.

DO THE EXERCISE
Inhale and slowly extend your right leg behind you, keeping it straight. At the same time, bend forward at the hip. Ideally, you should get to the point where a straight line, parallel to the floor, runs from your foot to your head, with the weight hanging directly below your shoulder. Slowly return to the starting position as you exhale. Do Arrows on your left leg for 30 seconds, then on your right leg for 30 seconds.

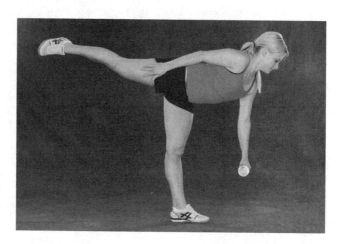

Hollywood Hamstring Curl

This is an amazingly efficient way to work your hamstrings using nothing more than your own body weight.

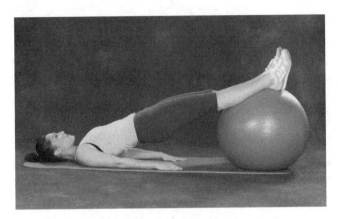

GET READY

Lie back on the floor with your heels on a stability ball. Raise your hips up so that your body forms a straight line from your shoulders to your feet. You can place your arms underneath yourself to help with balance.

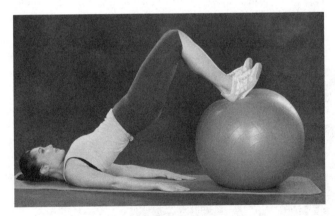

DO THE EXERCISE

Take a deep breath. Exhale and slowly draw the ball in toward your thighs by bending your knees. Try to keep your hips up the entire time, as if your body can't bend at the hips or the waist. When your knees are at a 45-degree angle, hold for a beat, then slowly let the ball roll back out to the starting position as you inhale, keeping your hips raised.

Hollywood Zorro Lunge

It's like fencing without a sword. This lunge variation will work almost your entire lower body, and the unique positioning of your feet will give you a nice stretch on the inside of your thighs.

GET READY

Stand with your feet together and your toes angled out at 45 degrees. Your hands should be on your hips.

DO THE EXERCISE

Inhale and step deeply out at a 45-degree angle—the direction your toe was pointing—with your right foot. Just as when doing squats, you want to make sure your knee stays over your heel or over the middle of your foot. Pretend to do a sword attack with your right hand if you want to. This makes the exercise more fun. Hold this position for a beat, then return to the starting position by driving off the right foot as you exhale. Repeat, this time lunging with the left foot.

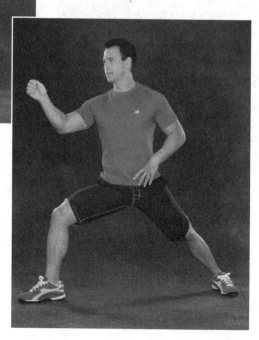

Hollywood Side Raise

This exercise tones and strengthens the muscles that make up the outer edges of your buttocks. The interesting rotation of the hip will give you a nice stretch that you'll feel in your glutes.

GET READY
Stand with your feet slightly closer than hip-width apart and your hands on your hips.

DO THE EXERCISE
Turn your right foot inward a little. Your toes, which had been facing forward, should now be facing to the left slightly. Take a deep breath. Exhale and slowly raise your leg out to the side, keeping your leg straight and your ankle bent at a 90-degree angle. When your leg is about 45 degrees off the floor, hold for a beat, then return to the starting position as you inhale. Do 30 seconds of raises with your right leg, then 30 seconds with your left leg.

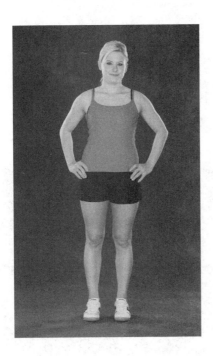 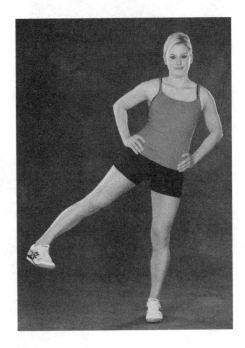

Hollywood Squeeze Play

The muscles of the inner thigh can be tough to work. This is an easy and super-efficient way to get the job done.

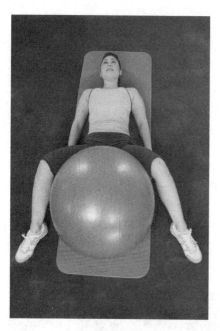

GET READY
Lie back with your knees bent and a stability ball between your legs.

DO THE EXERCISE
Take a deep breath. Exhale and squeeze the ball as tightly as you can with your thighs. Hold for a five-count, then loosen your grip as you inhale.

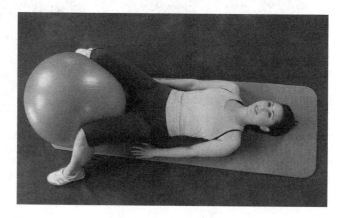

Celebrity Abs

Take a look at the magazines on the store shelves, and you'll see that almost all of them have one thing in common. I don't care whether it's a gossip magazine, a music magazine, a sports magazine, or a fitness magazine—the odds are, what's going to be staring up at you from the cover is a ripped set of abs.

We're a six pack–obsessed people, but very few people know how to get them. There are two keys. You have to make sure that the ab muscles are strong. And, more important, you have to get rid of the body fat that's covering them.

Strengthening the muscles that make up the abs is easy; they have very little range of motion. My strategy makes it even easier. Think of the abs as four distinct parts: the upper abs, the middle abs, the lower abs, and the outer abs. I've discovered that if you train the lower abs and the outer abs, you'll end up working the upper and middle abs at the same time. This doesn't work the other way around, though. If you concentrate on the upper abs, the lower abs won't benefit. By realizing this, I've streamlined ab training and made it about as efficient and effective as it can get.

After we know that the ab muscles are strong enough, all we have to do is get rid of the body fat that's blocking them from the public eye. This second part of the equation is really what this entire program is all about: building lean muscle to increase your metabolism and day-to-day calorie burn, doing cardio to blaze through the calories in large chunks, and following a nutrition program that's going to fuel your body in a way that will force you to burn body fat when you exercise.

With both bases covered, you're now officially a six-pack just waiting to happen.

Ab Muscles

The rectus abdominus is the muscle that we commonly refer to as the abs, although you'll see that while it may be the major player, your abs aren't a one-man show. Pound for pound, this muscle gets more press and attention than any other in the body. The actual muscle is only about the thickness of a quarter and about the height and the width of a magazine. It runs from the pubic bone to various points along the rib cage. Its job is to draw the rib cage toward the pelvis. Compared to the other muscles in the body, its job is actually very boring. The six-pack look is created by tendonous strips that cut across the muscle, dividing it into eight sections. In theory, you could get an eight-pack, but you'd need to get your body fat percentage so low that you'd probably be too weak to show off your ultra-ripped midsection. Besides, in many of us, those two lowest sections are covered with connective tissue that would prevent them from ever showing.

The external obliques are the muscles that run diagonally down toward your lower abdomen from the base of your rib cage. The job of the obliques is to help you move laterally at the hips—bending to your side, for example—and to twist the upper body. Well-developed obliques frame the rectus abdominus and help to create a complete package look to the abs.

Hollywood Crunch

This is similar to a traditional crunch but gives you a lot more bang for your buck. Instead of just targeting the middle and upper abs as a regular crunch does, here we'll hit the lower abs, too. The key is to get your hips up off the floor. I really want you to use some of the stability techniques that I talked about in chapter 2 here. It's very important to create that cylinder of power that connects your upper body with your lower body when you're doing core work, so remember—take a deep breath into your lower abdomen and then pull your belly button in toward your spine before you begin. You also want to make sure your neck is safe during your ab work. Pressing the tip of your tongue against the inside of your top upper teeth will add a lot of stability to your neck. You still want to make sure that you're not yanking your chin into your chest with every crunch, though. Maintain a space between your chin and your chest throughout the exercise. Crossing your hands in front of your chest is a great way to avoid potential neck pain. You can keep your hands behind your head if you want, but remember, they're there to offer light support to your head, not to slowly and methodically tear it off.

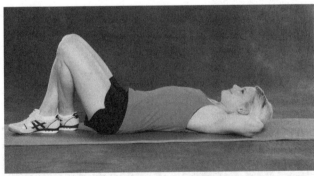

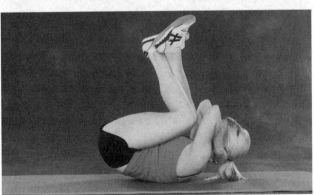

GET READY

Lie back on the floor with your hands either behind your head or crossed in front of your shoulders. Your knees should be bent and both feet should be flat on the floor.

DO THE EXERCISE

Take a deep breath. Exhale and slowly curl forward with your upper body until your shoulder blades come off the ground. At the same time, slowly lift your hips and bring your knees up toward your head. Hold this contraction for a beat, then return to the starting position as you inhale.

One-Legged Hollywood Crunch

This is a variation on the Hollywood Crunch that you'll definitely feel in your lower abs and in the muscles on the front side of your hips.

GET READY

Begin from an almost identical position as in the Hollywood Crunch but with one big exception: instead of bending your knees and your feet being flat on the floor, your legs are straight and they're pointing straight up at the ceiling.

DO THE EXERCISE

Take a deep breath. As in the Hollywood Crunch, begin by exhaling and slowly lifting your shoulder blades off the floor, making sure to keep your chin up. At the same time, lower your right knee toward your chest. This will raise your hips up off the floor. Hold this contraction for a beat and return to the starting position as you inhale. Repeat, this time bringing your left knee down toward your chest.

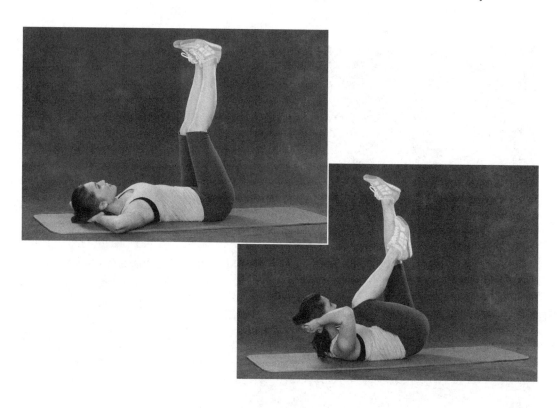

Hollywood Crossover Crunch

Here's a third crunch variation that again targets the upper, middle, and lower abs. As a bonus, because of the position of the leg, this is a great stretch for the hips and the butt.

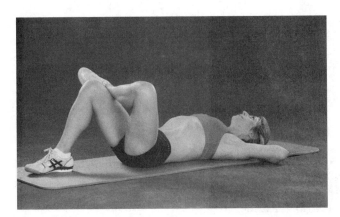

GET READY

Lie back on the floor with your hands behind your head, lightly supporting it. Your knees should be bent and both feet should be flat on the floor. Cross your legs so that the outside of your left ankle rests against your right knee.

DO THE EXERCISE

Take a deep breath. Exhale and slowly curl forward with your upper body until your shoulder blades come off the ground. At the same time, slowly lift your hips and bring your knees up toward your head. Hold this contraction for a beat, then return to the starting position as you inhale. Repeat for 30 seconds with the left leg crossed, then switch legs for the remaining 30 seconds.

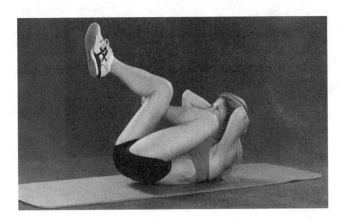

Hollywood Ball Small Sit-Up

Here are some more crunches, this time on a stability ball. Stabilizing your body while exercising on the ball forces your glutes, hamstrings, and calves to play along as you strengthen your abs.

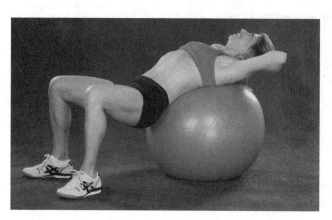

GET READY

Sit on top of the ball with your feet flat on the floor and slightly wider than hip-width apart. Slowly walk your feet out and roll down the ball until it is under and supporting your lower back. You can have your hands either behind your head, gently supporting it, or crossed in front of your chest.

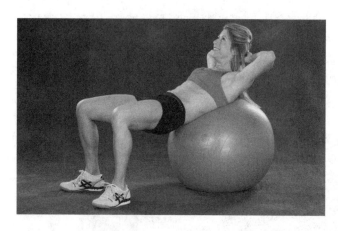

DO THE EXERCISE

Take a deep breath. Exhale and slowly raise your upper body, making sure to keep your head from bobbing forward. Remember to keep that space between your chin and your chest. Come up until you can feel a contraction in your abs. Hold the position for a beat, then return to the starting position as you inhale.

Pedal Your Waist Away

This is a twisting crunch that targets the entire abdominal area. The reason I'm smiling in the picture is that I only had to do five of them.

GET READY

Lie back on the floor with your hands behind your head, gently supporting it. Raise your legs off the floor at a 45-degree angle, keeping them straight. If this is too difficult, you can do the exercise starting with your knees bent and both feet flat on the floor.

DO THE EXERCISE

Take a deep breath. Exhale and slowly lift your right shoulder blade off the floor while twisting your upper body to the left. At the same time, draw your left knee in—raising your hips off the floor—and twist your lower body to the right. Hold this position, with your left knee and right elbow close to each other, for a beat. Return to the starting position as you inhale, and repeat with your left elbow and right knee.

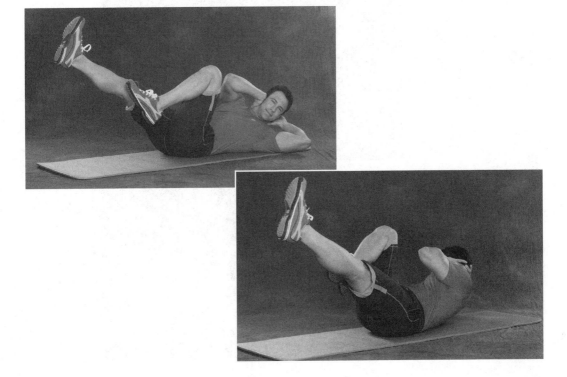

Hollywood Reaching Penguins

This is a great exercise for all parts of the abs and the obliques.

GET READY

Lie back with your hips and knees bent at 90-degree angles and your hips slightly raised off the floor. Raise your shoulder blades off the floor. Your arms should be by your sides and slightly off the floor.

DO THE EXERCISE

Take a deep breath. Exhale and slowly reach your right hand down toward your right ankle by bending your body to the right. Slowly return as you inhale. Then exhale and try to touch your left hand to your left ankle by bending your body to the left. Keep your hips, shoulder blades, and arms off the floor for the entire exercise if you can. If you're having trouble, do the exercise from a bent-knee position with both feet flat on the floor.

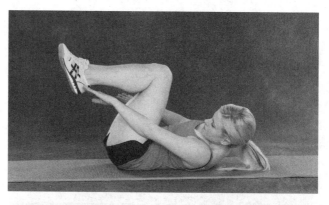

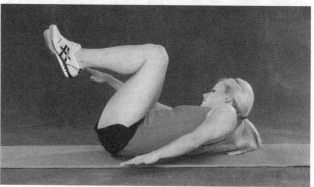

Hollywood Ball Crunch

This is one of the rare ab exercises done face down as opposed to face up. This is a full-body exercise. You'll build strength and stability in the shoulders, hips, and legs, but the centerpiece, what's holding the motion together, is your abs.

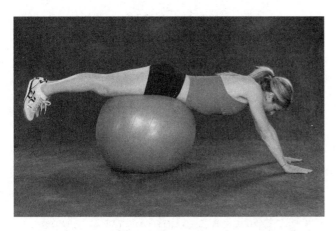

GET READY

Drape yourself over a stability ball and, keeping your body straight, walk your hands forward until you are in a push-up position with the ball resting under and slightly between your thighs.

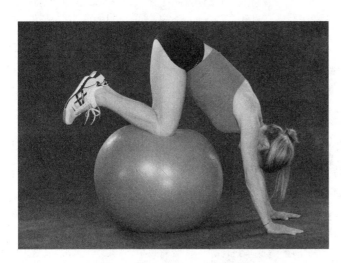

DO THE EXERCISE

Take a deep breath. Exhale and slowly bring your knees toward your chest. Your butt will raise and point toward the ceiling as the ball rolls forward and comes to rest under your shins. Inhale and slowly let the ball roll back to the starting position by lowering your butt and straightening your body.

Hollywood Leg Lift

Remember what I said about targeting the lower abs. This exercise does just that. If you're not sure what it feels like to work your lower abs, you will after a few of these. You want to make sure that you raise your hips up off the floor to get the most from the motion.

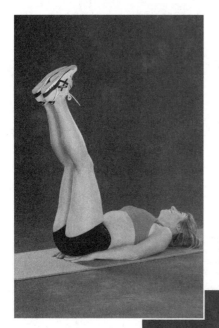

GET READY

Lie back with your hips bent at a 90-degree angle and your legs straight up. You can place your hands under your butt if you want to; some people find that this takes pressure off their lower backs.

DO THE EXERCISE

Take a deep breath. Exhale and very slowly raise your hips off the floor, keeping your legs straight and pointed straight up. The key is to go slowly and with great control. Imagine that you're trying to leave two footprints on the ceiling. Hold for a beat and slowly lower yourself to the starting position as you inhale.

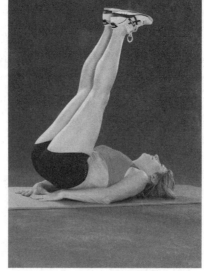

Hollywood Corkscrew

This is a challenging exercise that will not only work the obliques but will also strengthen your lower back, chest, and shoulders.

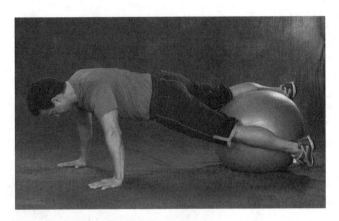

GET READY

Drape yourself over a stability ball and slowly walk yourself out into a push-up position. Keep your arms straight, with your elbows locked out, and your body straight throughout the exercise. Slide your feet down alongside the ball until you can squeeze it between your feet. Go slowly on this one.

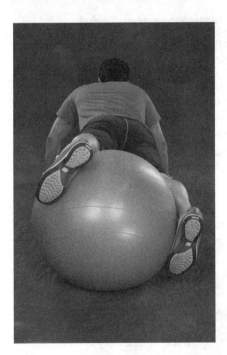

DO THE EXERCISE

Take a deep breath. Exhale and slowly lower your right foot toward the floor. This will cause your left hip to rise. Lower your foot to within about an inch of the floor, then slowly rotate your lower body back to the starting position as you inhale. Repeat on the other side.

Hollywood Surfboard with Alternating Leg Lifts

This is another abs exercise designed to work your lower back as well.

GET READY

Assume an up push-up position, but instead of having your hands on the floor, support yourself on your forearms. Have your elbows positioned directly below your shoulders.

DO THE EXERCISE

Take a deep breath. Exhale and, keeping your leg straight, slowly lift your left foot about a foot off the ground. Keep your body as rigid as possible and try not to raise your butt toward the ceiling. Hold for a five-count and inhale as you lower yourself to the starting position. Continue, alternating legs and holding each position for a five-count.

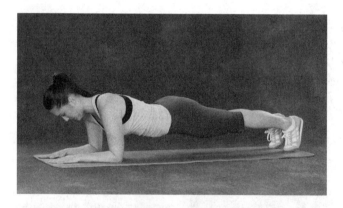

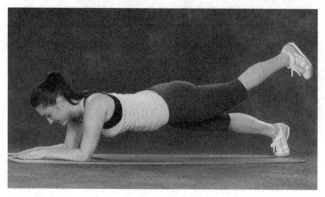

Side Plank with Hollywood Hip Raise

If your abs were the centerpiece of the full-body Hollywood Ball Crunch, your obliques, the muscles along the sides of your midsection, are the stars of this full-body exercise. In addition to working your core, you'll also be strengthening the stabilizers in your shoulders and improving your overall sense of balance.

GET READY

Lie on your left side with your right leg stacked on top of your left leg and your left elbow directly under your left shoulder.

DO THE EXERCISE

Take a deep breath. Exhale and slowly press your hips up toward the ceiling. When your body is perfectly straight from your heels to the top of your head, hold the position for a five-count, then lower yourself back to the starting position as you inhale. Do 30 seconds of raises on your left side, then 30 seconds on your right side.

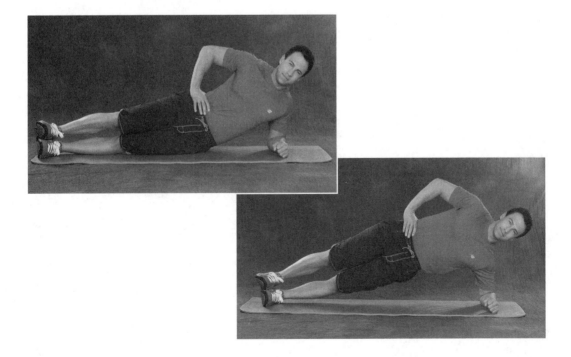

7

The Celebrity Makeover Walking Phase— Weeks 1 and 2

The first phase of my program is designed to ease your body into fitness. All of this may be new to you, so I want to get your body used to working out gradually. Every workout is broken down into segments, alternating periods of cardio and strength training. In this first phase, the cardio you'll do is walking in place. You'll do your cardio—for now, walking—for 2 minutes, then immediately switch to a strength exercise for 1 minute, then quickly back to your walking, and so on. It's designed to get—and keep—your heart rate up. And it will.

When you're finished with each exercise, I want you to carefully put the dumbbells down on the floor or on a small table before starting to walk. This will help the muscles you've just worked recover and be ready to go when it's time to exercise them again.

Why Walking?

I want your cardio for the initial phase of my program to be something that I don't have to go into much detail about and that you

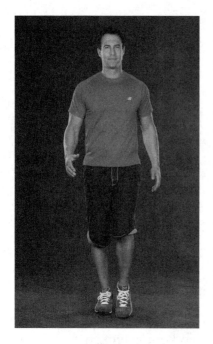

don't have to do much thinking about. Walking fits the bill perfectly. Most of us have been walking since before we can remember.

But I'm not just having you walk because I know you can do it. Walking is a great way to get the heart rate up and burn calories without too much effort. Studies have shown that people who simply walk on a regular basis outlive their more sedentary peers. Just by walking. Think about that.

Walking is also a great way to get your whole body moving in sync. When you walk, you do more than just move your legs. The swinging of your arms that coincides with the movement of your legs helps to balance your entire body.

Before you start, read through some of the workouts to familiarize yourself with the strength exercises. The descriptions of all the motions are in chapter 6, "Celebrity Makeover Exercises," so be sure to check there to make sure you're doing things correctly.

If at any time you feel tired, take a break. Listen to your body. These first two weeks are about transitioning you into a new and healthier lifestyle. I want to get your body used to exercising gradually. I'm not here to destroy you. All I ask is that you do your best.

The Initiation Phase

I like to call the nutrition portion of the first two weeks of my program the initiation phase. It's almost like a detoxifying period for your body. You'll be eating very cleanly and healthfully. Coupled with the exercise, it's designed to let you see real results quickly. And you will, if you follow these rules:

- For your three main meals and three booster meals, you can choose only from primary proteins and primary carbohydrates (see chapter 4).

- Do not drink any alcoholic beverages.

- Have caffeine in very limited amounts.

- Don't eat for 1½ hours before working out. If you train first thing in the morning, refer back to chapter 4 for my breakfast suggestions.

Don't worry, it's not as hard as it sounds. And the good news is that after these first two weeks, you'll get a more varied choice of what to eat in the introduction phase. By the time you get into my regular nutrition plan, you'll feel as if you're at an all-you-can-eat buffet. Well, almost.

Walking Workout—Week One, Workout One

- Cleansing Minute (see pages 73–74)
- Walking—2 minutes
- Hollywood Butt Kick—1 minute (see page 121)
- Walking—2 minutes
- Hollywood Squeeze Play—1 minute (see page 126)
- Walking—2 minutes
- Hollywood Sumo Squat with Calf Raise—1 minute (see page 120)
- Walking—2 minutes
- Beginner Push-Up—1 minute (see page 84)
- Walking—2 minutes
- Hollywood Kickback with a Twist—1 minute (see page 110)
- Walking—2 minutes
- Hollywood One-Armed Row—1 minute (see page 93)
- Walking—2 minutes
- Hollywood Bent-Over Rear Delt—1 minute (see page 103)
- Walking—2 minutes
- Hollywood Surfboard with Alternating Leg Lifts—1 minute (see page 138)
- Rest—30 seconds
- Hollywood Crunch—1 minute (see page 129)
- Rest—30 seconds
- Hollywood Crossover Crunch—1 minute (see page 131)
- Walking—2 minutes

- Cleansing Minute (see pages 73–74)
- Walking—2 minutes
- Hollywood W Shoulders—1 minute (see page 100)
- Walking—2 minutes
- Push-Ups (Beginner or Intermediate)—1 minute (see page 84–85)
- Walking—2 minutes
- Hollywood Kickback with a Twist—1 minute (see page 110)
- Walking—2 minutes
- Hollywood Bent-Over Row—1 minute (see page 94)
- Walking—2 minutes
- Hollywood Hammer Curl—1 minute (see page 107)
- Walking—2 minutes
- Hollywood Sumo Squat with Calf Raise—1 minute (see page 120)
- Walking—2 minutes
- Hollywood Hamstring Curl—1 minute (see page 123)
- Walking—2 minutes
- Hollywood Reaching Penguins—1 minute (see page 134)
- Rest—30 seconds
- Hollywood Crunch—1 minute (see page 129)
- Rest—30 seconds
- Side Plank with Hollywood Hip Raise—1 minute (see page 139)
- Walking—2 minutes

Walking Workout—Week One, Workout Two

- Cleansing Minute (see pages 73–74)
- Walking—2 minutes
- Hollywood Bent-Over Rear Delt—1 minute (see page 103)
- Walking—2 minutes
- Hollywood One-Armed Row—1 minute (see page 93)
- Walking—2 minutes
- Hollywood Incline Fly—1 minute (see page 88)
- Walking—2 minutes
- Hollywood Kickback with a Twist—1 minute (see page 110)
- Walking—2 minutes
- Biceps Curl with a Hollywood Twist—1 minute (see page 106)
- Walking—2 minutes
- Hollywood Hamstring Curl—1 minute (see page 123)
- Walking—2 minutes
- Hollywood "I Dream of Jeannie" Squat—1 minute (see page 119)
- Walking—2 minutes
- Hollywood Reaching Penguins—1 minute (see page 134)
- Rest—30 seconds
- Hollywood Surfboard with Alternating Leg Lifts—1 minute (see page 138)
- Rest—30 seconds
- Pedal Your Waist Away—1 minute (see page 133)
- Walking—2 minutes

- Cleansing Minute (see pages 73–74)

- Walking—2 minutes

- Push-Ups (Beginner or Intermediate)—1 minute (see pages 84–85)

- Walking—2 minutes

- Hollywood Bent-Over Row—1 minute (see page 94)

- Walking—2 minutes

- Hollywood Kickback with a Twist—1 minute (see page 110)

- Walking—2 minutes

- Hollywood W Shoulders—1 minute (see page 100)

- Walking—2 minutes

- Hollywood Hammer Curl—1 minute (see page 107)

- Walking—2 minutes

- Hollywood Hamstring Curl—1 minute (see page 123)

- Walking—2 minutes

- Hollywood Sumo Squat with Calf Raise—1 minute (see page 120)

- Walking—2 minutes

- Hollywood Surfboard with Alternating Leg Lifts—1 minute (see page 138)

- Rest—30 seconds

- Side Plank with Hollywood Hip Raise—1 minute (see page 139)

- Rest—30 seconds

- Hollywood Crossover Crunch—1 minute (see page 131)

- Walking—2 minutes

Walking Workout—Week One, Workout Three

- Cleansing Minute (see pages 73–74)
- Walking—2 minutes
- Hollywood Sumo Squat with Calf Raise—1 minute (see page 120)
- Walking—2 minutes
- Hollywood Squeeze Play—1 minute (see page 126)
- Walking—2 minutes
- Hollywood Side Raise—1 minute (see page 125)
- Walking—2 minutes
- Hollywood One-Armed Row—1 minute (see page 93)
- Walking—2 minutes
- Hollywood Kickback with a Twist—1 minute (see page 110)
- Walking—2 minutes
- Hollywood Incline Fly—1 minute (see page 88)
- Walking—2 minutes
- Biceps Curl with a Hollywood Twist—1 minute (see page 106)
- Walking—2 minutes
- Hollywood Ball Small Sit-Up—1 minute (see page 132)
- Rest—30 seconds
- Pedal Your Waist Away—1 minute (see page 133)
- Rest—30 seconds
- Hollywood Crossover Crunch—1 minute (see page 131)
- Walking—2 minutes

- Cleansing Minute (see pages 73–74)
- Walking—2 minutes
- Hollywood"I Dream of Jeannie"Squat—1 minute (see page 119)
- Walking—2 minutes
- Hollywood Hamstring Curl—1 minute (see page 123)
- Walking—2 minutes
- Push-Ups (Beginner or Intermediate)—1 minute (see pages 84–85)
- Walking—2 minutes
- Hollywood Bent-Over Row—1 minute (see page 94)
- Walking—2 minutes
- Hollywood W Shoulders—1 minute (see page 100)
- Walking—2 minutes
- Hollywood Kickback with a Twist—1 minute (see page 110)
- Walking—2 minutes
- Hollywood Hammer Curl—1 minute (see page 107)
- Walking—2 minutes
- Pedal Your Waist Away—1 minute (see page 133)
- Rest—30 seconds
- Hollywood Crunch—1 minute (see page 129)
- Rest—30 seconds
- Hollywood Reaching Penguins—1 minute (see page 134)
- Walking—2 minutes

Walking Workout—Week Two, Workout One

- Cleansing Minute (see pages 73–74)
- Walking—2 minutes
- Hollywood Butt Kick—1 minute (see page 121)
- Walking—2 minutes
- Beginner Push-Up—1 minute (see page 84)
- Walking—2 minutes
- Hollywood Bent-Over Rear Delt—1 minute (see page 103)
- Walking—2 minutes
- Hollywood One-Armed Row—1 minute (see page 93)
- Walking—2 minutes
- Hollywood Kickback with a Twist—1 minute (see page 110)
- Walking—2 minutes
- Biceps Curl with a Hollywood Twist—1 minute (see page 106)
- Walking—2 minutes
- Hollywood Hamstring Curl—1 minute (see page 123)
- Walking—2 minutes
- Pedal Your Waist Away—1 minute (see page 133)
- Rest—30 seconds
- One-Legged Hollywood Crunch—1 minute (see page 130)
- Rest—30 seconds
- Hollywood Reaching Penguins—1 minute (see page 134)
- Walking—2 minutes

- Cleansing Minute (see pages 73–74)
- Walking—2 minutes
- Hollywood W Shoulders—1 minute (see page 100)
- Walking—2 minutes
- Hollywood Bent-Over Row—1 minute (see page 94)
- Walking—2 minutes
- Hollywood Incline Fly—1 minute (see page 88)
- Walking—2 minutes
- Hollywood Kickback with a Twist—1 minute (see page 110)
- Walking—2 minutes
- Hollywood Hammer Curl—1 minute (see page 107)
- Walking—2 minutes
- Hollywood Hamstring Curl—1 minute (see page 123)
- Walking—2 minutes
- Hollywood "I Dream of Jeannie" Squat—1 minute (see page 119)
- Walking—2 minutes
- Hollywood Leg Lift—1 minute (see page 136)
- Rest—30 seconds
- Side Plank with Hollywood Hip Raise—1 minute (see page 139)
- Rest—30 seconds
- Pedal Your Waist Away—1 minute (see page 133)
- Walking—2 minutes

Walking Workout—Week Two, Workout Two

Women

- Cleansing Minute (see pages 73–74)
- Walking—2 minutes
- Hollywood Squeeze Play—1 minute (see page 126)
- Walking—2 minutes
- Hollywood Butt Kick—1 minute (see page 121)
- Walking—2 minutes
- Beginner Push-Up—1 minute (see page 84)
- Walking—2 minutes
- Hollywood Bent-Over Rear Delt—1 minute (see page 103)
- Walking—2 minutes
- Hollywood Kickback with a Twist—1 minute (see page 110)
- Walking—2 minutes
- Hollywood One-Armed Row—1 minute (see page 93)
- Walking—2 minutes
- Biceps Curl with a Hollywood Twist—1 minute (see page 106)
- Walking—2 minutes
- Hollywood Surfboard with Alternating Leg Lifts—1 minute (see page 138)
- Rest—30 seconds
- Side Plank with Hollywood Hip Raise—1 minute (see page 139)
- Rest—30 seconds
- Pedal Your Waist Away—1 minute (see page 133)
- Walking—2 minutes

- Cleansing Minute (see pages 73–74)
- Walking—2 minutes
- Hollywood Sumo Squat with Calf Raise—1 minute (see page 120)
- Walking—2 minutes
- Hollywood Hamstring Curl—1 minute (see page 123)
- Walking—2 minutes
- Hollywood Kickback with a Twist—1 minute (see page 110)
- Walking—2 minutes
- Hollywood W Shoulders—1 minute (see page 100)
- Walking—2 minutes
- Hollywood Bent-Over Row—1 minute (see page 94)
- Walking—2 minutes
- Push-Ups (Beginner or Intermediate)—1 minute (see pages 84–85)
- Walking—2 minutes
- Hollywood Hammer Curl—1 minute (see page 107)
- Walking—2 minutes
- Hollywood Surfboard with Alternating Leg Lifts—1 minute (see page 138)
- Rest—30 seconds
- Hollywood Leg Lift—1 minute (see page 136)
- Rest—30 seconds
- Side Plank with Hollywood Hip Raise—1 minute (see page 139)
- Walking—2 minutes

Walking Workout—Week Two, Workout Three

- Cleansing Minute (see pages 73–74)
- Walking—2 minutes
- Hollywood Bent-Over Rear Delt—1 minute (see page 103)
- Walking—2 minutes
- Hollywood One-Armed Row—1 minute (see page 93)
- Walking—2 minutes
- Hollywood Kickback with a Twist—1 minute (see page 110)
- Walking—2 minutes
- Hollywood Incline Fly—1 minute (see page 88)
- Walking—2 minutes
- Biceps Curl with a Hollywood Twist—1 minute (see page 106)
- Walking—2 minutes
- Hollywood Hamstring Curl—1 minute (see page 123)
- Walking—2 minutes
- Hollywood Butt Kick—1 minute (see page 121)
- Walking—2 minutes
- Hollywood Leg Lift—1 minute (see page 136)
- Rest—30 seconds
- Hollywood Crunch—1 minute (see page 129)
- Rest—30 seconds
- Hollywood Surfboard with Alternating Leg Lifts—1 minute (see page 138)
- Walking—2 minutes

- Cleansing Minute (see pages 73–74)
- Walking—2 minutes
- Hollywood Kickback with a Twist—1 minute (see page 110)
- Walking—2 minutes
- Hollywood W Shoulders—1 minute (see page 100)
- Walking—2 minutes
- Hollywood Incline Fly—1 minute (see page 88)
- Walking—2 minutes
- Hollywood Bent-Over Row—1 minute (see page 94)
- Walking—2 minutes
- Hollywood Hammer Curl—1 minute (see page 107)
- Walking—2 minutes
- Hollywood "I Dream of Jeannie" Squat—1 minute (see page 119)
- Walking—2 minutes
- Hollywood Hamstring Curl—1 minute (see page 123)
- Walking—2 minutes
- Pedal Your Waist Away—1 minute (see page 133)
- Rest—30 seconds
- One-Legged Hollywood Crunch—1 minute (see page 130)
- Rest—30 seconds
- Hollywood Reaching Penguins—1 minute (see page 134)
- Walking—2 minutes

Two-Week Measurements

Neck _____ Shoulders _____

Chest _____ Waist _____ Hips _____

Right biceps (flexed) _____ Left biceps (flexed) _____

Right thigh _____ Left thigh _____

Right calf _____ Left calf _____

Resting heart rate _____

Body fat percentage _____

8

The Celebrity Makeover Marching Phase— Weeks 3 and 4

You're doing a great job, so far. If you're reading this page, it's because you successfully made it through the program's first two weeks. Congratulations. The first two weeks of any new program can often be the toughest: you have to change your daily routine to make time to exercise, you have to closely monitor what you eat and how much you sleep, and, in general, you need to be more aware of your health. You've made it past the first major hurdle!

In the second phase of the program, the cardio you'll do will switch to marching in place. It's a step up from walking in place, but if you've been giving it your all for the last two weeks, you should be able to handle it. Go slowly at first, and take a break when you need to.

Hup Two, Three, Four

Marching will hit your body a little bit harder than walking does. The marching I want you to do will have you bringing your knee up to waist height with each step. This strengthens the muscles in the front of the thigh, while also giving the muscles that extend the hip—your glutes—a slight stretch with each step. I want you to be keenly aware

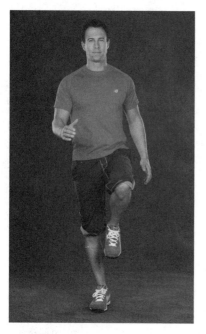

of your posture. Stand up a little bit straighter than you did during the walking phase and keep your chin up. This will force the muscles in the back, especially the erectors in your lower back, to do a little more work. As far as your tempo goes, march at a slightly faster pace than you did when walking. Remember, marching is done by soldiers, and they generally have someplace they're trying to get to. March with a purpose. This faster tempo will keep your heart rate up higher and help you to burn more calories. Regarding your strength training, I'll be introducing you to some new motions over the next two weeks. Flip through some of the workouts to see the new exercises, and then check chapter 6 to make sure you'll know how to do them.

Nutrition Update

There's some good news on the nutrition front. You're now entering the introduction phase of the nutrition plan. While you'll still be eating only primary proteins and carbs for half of your meals, you're now able to choose from the secondary lists of proteins and carbs for the rest of your meals and booster meals. Remember, if you choose a primary protein, you can have either twice as much of a primary carb or the same amount of a secondary carb. If you go with a secondary protein, you can have either the same-size portion of a primary carb or a half-size portion of a secondary carb. Check out my meal suggestions at the end of chapter 4 or feel free to use these guidelines and create your own delicious meals. And if you're still even a little bit confused about how my plan works, go back and reread the section about my nutrition program. I want things to be crystal clear to you so that you can make the smartest choices about what you eat and will be able to see the results you want faster.

Keep up the good work—only eight weeks left!

Marching Workout—Week Three, Workout One

Women

- Cleansing Minute (see pages 73–74)
- Marching—2 minutes
- Hollywood "I Dream of Jeannie" Squat—1 minute (see page 119)
- Marching—2 minutes
- Hollywood Squeeze Play—1 minute (see page 126)
- Marching—2 minutes
- Hollywood Butt Kick—1 minute (see page 121)
- Marching—2 minutes
- Hollywood Bent-Over Rear Delt—1 minute (see page 103)
- Marching—2 minutes
- Hollywood Overhead Tri—1 minute (see page 113)
- Marching—2 minutes
- Hollywood Bent-Over Row—1 minute (see page 94)
- Marching—2 minutes
- Hollywood Incline Fly—1 minute (see page 88)
- Marching—2 minutes
- Hollywood Surfboard with Alternating Leg Lifts—1 minute (see page 138)
- Rest—30 seconds
- Side Plank with Hollywood Hip Raise—1 minute (see page 139)
- Rest—30 seconds
- Hollywood Leg Lift—1 minute (see page 136)
- Marching—2 minutes

- Cleansing Minute (see pages 73–74)
- Marching—2 minutes
- Hollywood "I Dream of Jeannie" Squat—1 minute (see page 119)
- Marching—2 minutes
- Hollywood Hamstring Curl—1 minute (see page 123)
- Marching—2 minutes
- Hollywood Fly—1 minute (see page 87)
- Marching—2 minutes
- Hollywood One-Armed Row—1 minute (see page 93)
- Marching—2 minutes
- Hollywood Bent-Over Rear Delt—1 minute (see page 103)
- Marching—2 minutes
- Hollywood Overhead Tri—1 minute (see page 113)
- Marching—2 minutes
- Biceps Curl with a Hollywood Twist—1 minute (see page 110)
- Marching—2 minutes
- Pedal Your Waist Away—1 minute (see page 133)
- Rest—30 seconds
- One-Legged Hollywood Crunch—1 minute (see page 130)
- Rest—30 seconds
- Hollywood Reaching Penguins—1 minute (see page 134)
- Marching—2 minutes

Marching Workout—Week Three, Workout Two

- Cleansing Minute (see pages 73–74)
- Marching—2 minutes
- Hollywood Kickback with a Twist—1 minute (see page 110)
- Marching—2 minutes
- Hollywood W Shoulders—1 minute (see page 100)
- Marching—2 minutes
- Hollywood Fly—1 minute (see page 87)
- Marching—2 minutes
- Hollywood One-Armed Row—1 minute (see page 93)
- Marching—2 minutes
- Hollywood Sumo Squat with Calf Raise—1 minute (see page 120)
- Marching—2 minutes
- Hollywood Butt Kick—1 minute (see page 121)
- Marching—2 minutes
- Hollywood Side Raise—1 minute (see page 125)
- Marching—2 minutes
- Pedal Your Waist Away—1 minute (see page 133)
- Rest—30 seconds
- Side Plank with Hollywood Hip Raise—1 minute (see page 139)
- Rest—30 seconds
- Hollywood Ball Small Sit-Up—1 minute (see page 132)
- Marching—2 minutes

- Cleansing Minute (see pages 73–74)
- Marching—2 minutes
- Hollywood W Shoulders—1 minute (see page 100)
- Marching—2 minutes
- Hollywood Bent-Over Row—1 minute (see page 94)
- Marching—2 minutes
- Hollywood Incline Fly—1 minute (see page 88)
- Marching—2 minutes
- Hollywood Kickback with a Twist—1 minute (see page 110)
- Marching—2 minutes
- Hollywood Hammer Curl—1 minute (see page 107)
- Marching—2 minutes
- Hollywood "I Dream of Jeannie" Squat—1 minute (see page 119)
- Marching—2 minutes
- Hollywood Hamstring Curl—1 minute (see page 123)
- Marching—2 minutes
- Hollywood Surfboard with Alternating Leg Lifts—1 minute (see page 138)
- Rest—30 seconds
- Side Plank with Hollywood Hip Raise—1 minute (see page 139)
- Rest—30 seconds
- Pedal Your Waist Away—1 minute (see page 133)
- Marching—2 minutes

Marching Workout—Week Three, Workout Three

- Cleansing Minute (see pages 73–74)
- Marching—2 minutes
- Hollywood "I Dream of Jeannie" Squat—1 minute (see page 119)
- Marching—2 minutes
- Hollywood Hamstring Curl—1 minute (see page 123)
- Marching—2 minutes
- Push-Ups (Beginner or Intermediate)—1 minute (see pages 84–85)
- Marching—2 minutes
- Hollywood Bent-Over Row—1 minute (see page 94)
- Marching—2 minutes
- Hollywood Bent-Over Rear Delt—1 minute (see page 103)
- Marching—2 minutes
- Hollywood Overhead Tri—1 minute (see page 113)
- Marching—2 minutes
- Hollywood Hammer Curl—1 minute (see page 104)
- Marching—2 minutes
- Hollywood Reaching Penguins—1 minute (see page 134)
- Rest—30 seconds
- Hollywood Crunch—1 minute (see page 129)
- Rest—30 seconds
- Side Plank with Hollywood Hip Raise—1 minute (see page 139)
- Marching—2 minutes

- Cleansing Minute (see pages 73–74)

- Marching—2 minutes

- Hollywood Sumo Squat with Calf Raise—1 minute (see page 120)

- Marching—2 minutes

- Hollywood Hamstring Curl—1 minute (see page 123)

- Marching—2 minutes

- Push-Ups (Beginner or Intermediate)—1 minute (see pages 84–85)

- Marching—2 minutes

- Hollywood One-Armed Row—1 minute (see page 93)

- Marching—2 minutes

- Hollywood Bent-Over Rear Delt—1 minute (see page 103)

- Marching—2 minutes

- Hollywood Overhead Tri—1 minute (see page 113)

- Marching—2 minutes

- Hollywood Hammer Curl—1 minute (see page 107)

- Marching—2 minutes

- Hollywood Ball Small Sit-Up—1 minute (see page 132)

- Rest—30 seconds

- Hollywood Leg Lift—1 minute (see page 134)

- Rest—30 seconds

- Side Plank with Hollywood Hip Raise—1 minute (see page 139)

- Marching—2 minutes

Marching Workout—Week Four, Workout One

Women

- Cleansing Minute (see pages 73–74)
- Marching—2 minutes
- Hollywood Squeeze Play—1 minute (see page 126)
- Marching—2 minutes
- Hollywood Hamstring Curl—1 minute (see page 123)
- Marching—2 minutes
- Hollywood "I Dream of Jeannie" Squat—1 minute (see page 119)
- Marching—2 minutes
- Hollywood Incline Fly—1 minute (see page 88)
- Marching—2 minutes
- Hollywood W Shoulders—1 minute (see page 100)
- Marching—2 minutes
- Hollywood Overhead Tri—1 minute (see page 113)
- Marching—2 minutes
- Hollywood Hammer Curl—1 minute (see page 107)
- Marching—2 minutes
- Hollywood Ball Small Sit-Up—1 minute (see page 132)
- Rest—30 seconds
- Hollywood Surfboard with Alternating Leg Lifts—1 minute (see page 138)
- Rest—30 seconds
- Side Plank with Hollywood Hip Raise—1 minute (see page 139)
- Marching—2 minutes

- Cleansing Minute (see pages 73–74)
- Marching—2 minutes
- Push-Ups (Beginner or Intermediate)—1 minute (see pages 84–85)
- Marching—2 minutes
- Hollywood Bent-Over Row—1 minute (see page 94)
- Marching—2 minutes
- Hollywood W Shoulders—1 minute (see page 100)
- Marching—2 minutes
- Hollywood Kickback with a Twist—1 minute (see page 110)
- Marching—2 minutes
- Biceps Curl with a Hollywood Twist—1 minute (see page 106)
- Marching—2 minutes
- Hollywood Hamstring Curl—1 minute (see page 123)
- Marching—2 minutes
- Hollywood Sumo Squat with Calf Raise—1 minute (see page 120)
- Marching—2 minutes
- Hollywood Reaching Penguins—1 minute (see page 134)
- Rest—30 seconds
- Hollywood Crossover Crunch—1 minute (see page 131)
- Rest—30 seconds
- Hollywood Surfboard with Alternating Leg Lifts—1 minute (see page 138)
- Marching—2 minutes

Marching Workout—Week Four, Workout Two

Women

- Cleansing Minute (see pages 73–74)
- Marching—2 minutes
- Hollywood Butt Kick—1 minute (see pages 121)
- Marching—2 minutes
- Hollywood "I Dream of Jeannie" Squat—1 minute (see page 119)
- Marching—2 minutes
- Hollywood Squeeze Play—1 minute (see page 126)
- Marching—2 minutes
- Hollywood Bent-Over Rear Delt—1 minute (see page 103)
- Marching—2 minutes
- Hollywood Kickback with a Twist—1 minute (see page 110)
- Marching—2 minutes
- Hollywood Bent-Over Row—1 minute (see page 94)
- Marching—2 minutes
- Biceps Curl with a Hollywood Twist—1 minute (see page 106)
- Marching—2 minutes
- Hollywood Surfboard with Alternating Leg Lifts—1 minute (see page 138)
- Rest—30 seconds
- Side Plank with Hollywood Hip Raise—1 minute (see page 139)
- Rest—30 seconds
- Hollywood Crossover Crunch—1 minute (see page 131)
- Marching—2 minutes

- Cleansing Minute (see pages 73–74)
- Marching—2 minutes
- Hollywood Overhead Tri—1 minute (see page 113)
- Marching—2 minutes
- Hollywood Fly—1 minute (see page 87)
- Marching—2 minutes
- Hollywood One-Armed Row—1 minute (see page 93)
- Marching—2 minutes
- Hollywood Bent-Over Rear Delt—1 minute (see page 103)
- Marching—2 minutes
- Hollywood Hammer Curl—1 minute (see page 107)
- Marching—2 minutes
- Hollywood "I Dream of Jeannie" Squat—1 minute (see page 119)
- Marching—2 minutes
- Hollywood Hamstring Curl—1 minute (see page 123)
- Marching—2 minutes
- Hollywood Surfboard with Alternating Leg Lifts—1 minute (see page 138)
- Rest—30 seconds
- Side Plank with Hollywood Hip Raise—1 minute (see page 139)
- Rest—30 seconds
- Hollywood Leg Lift—1 minute (see page 136)
- Marching—2 minutes

Marching Workout—Week Four, Workout Three

Women

- Cleansing Minute (see pages 73–74)
- Marching—2 minutes
- Hollywood Kickback with a Twist—1 minute (see page 110)
- Marching—2 minutes
- Hollywood Bent-Over Rear Delt—1 minute (see page 103)
- Marching—2 minutes
- Hollywood Incline Fly—1 minute (see page 88)
- Marching—2 minutes
- Hollywood Bent-Over Row—1 minute (see page 94)
- Marching—2 minutes
- Hollywood Butt Kick—1 minute (see page 121)
- Marching—2 minutes
- Hollywood Sumo Squat with Calf Raise—1 minute (see page 120)
- Marching—2 minutes
- Hollywood Hamstring Curl—1 minute (see page 123)
- Marching—2 minutes
- Hollywood Corkscrew—1 minute (see page 137)
- Rest—30 seconds
- Pedal Your Waist Away—1 minute (see page 133)
- Rest—30 seconds
- Hollywood Reaching Penguins—1 minute (see page 134)
- Marching—2 minutes

- Cleansing Minute (see pages 73–74)
- Marching—2 minutes
- Hollywood Hamstring Curl—1 minute (see page 123)
- Marching—2 minutes
- Hollywood "I Dream of Jeannie" Squat—1 minute (see page 119)
- Marching—2 minutes
- Hollywood Incline Fly—1 minute (see page 88)
- Marching—2 minutes
- Hollywood Bent-Over Row—1 minute (see page 94)
- Marching—2 minutes
- Hollywood Overhead Tri—1 minute (see page 113)
- Marching—2 minutes
- Hollywood W Shoulders—1 minute (see page 100)
- Marching—2 minutes
- Biceps Curl with a Hollywood Twist—1 minute (see page 106)
- Marching—2 minutes
- Pedal Your Waist Away—1 minute (see page 133)
- Rest—30 seconds
- Hollywood Crunch—1 minute (see page 129)
- Rest—30 seconds
- Hollywood Ball Small Sit-Up—1 minute (see page 132)
- Marching—2 minutes

Four-Week Measurements

Neck _____ Shoulders _____

Chest _____ Waist _____ Hips _____

Right biceps (flexed) _____ Left biceps (flexed) _____

Right thigh _____ Left thigh _____

Right calf _____ Left calf _____

Resting heart rate _____

Body fat percentage _____

9

The Celebrity Makeover Jogging Phase— Weeks 5 and 6

'll bet it seems like only yesterday that you started my program, but when you finish this third phase, you'll be 60 percent through!

Cardio-wise, we're kicking things up a notch—a big notch. No more marching in place; now you're going to be jogging in place. It's a slightly faster pace, but we've been building up slowly so you should be ready. If you have trouble, you can slow it down, take a break, or even go back to marching in place for a while. I just want you to do your best.

Jogging

Jogging won't be as tough on the muscles in the front of your thigh, your hip flexors, as marching was, but the motion—the constant bouncing on the balls of your feet—will really work your calves. Working your calves this way dynamically and explosively for long periods at a time, in addition to the straight weight training we're already doing for them, will do more than just tone the muscles in the lower part of your leg; it will actually help to keep you young. You know how it's said that as people get older they lose the spring in

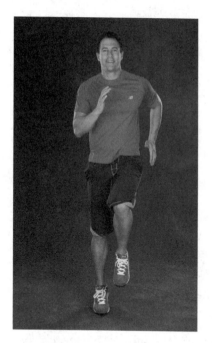

their step? Well, it's not just a polite or flowery way to talk about the aging process—it's true. As we get older, we lose strength in the calf muscles, both the gastrocnemius and the soleus. When this happens, we begin to walk differently. We shuffle our feet. We walk flat-footed. Jogging builds great strength in the calf muscles. As a result of having strong calf muscles, every step we take has a slight bounce to it: a spring in each step. Jogging is a surefire way to make certain that you never lose that. It's also a surefire way to burn a whole mess of calories in a short time. Just as marching increased the calorie burn over walking, jogging increases the number of calories you'll burn compared to those you burned marching.

Keep Track

Don't forget to monitor your stats. You should be on your third set of measurements by now. At this point, women should start to see reductions in the hip, waist, and thigh measurements. The numbers for the biceps might be the same, but I'll bet your arms feel a lot more solid these days and look a lot more toned. Men should start to see the measurements for the waist go down, while those for the chest, the biceps, and the thighs creep up as you strip away the fat from your midsection and add muscle to your torso, arms, and legs. Both women and men should see a change in their body fat percentage numbers and, depending on your physical condition when you started the program, you may have noticed that your resting heart rate has dropped by a beat or two.

Nutrition Update

You've completed the initiation and the introduction phases. Great job! That took a lot of willpower and self-discipline. As a reward, you're now able to take full advantage of my complete nutrition program. Try as much as possible to stick with primary proteins and primary carbs, but you're free to choose from the secondary list whenever you want. Remember, if you go with a primary protein, you can have twice as much of a primary carb or the same amount of a secondary carb. If you go with a secondary protein, you can have the same-size portion of a primary carb or a half-size portion of a secondary carb.

So far, so good. Just six weeks left!

Jogging Workout—Week Five, Workout One

Women

- Cleansing Minute (see pages 73–74)
- Jogging—2 minutes
- Hollywood Arrow—1 minute (see page 122)
- Jogging—2 minutes
- Hollywood Side Raise—1 minute (see page 125)
- Jogging—2 minutes
- Hollywood Squeeze Play—1 minute (see page 126)
- Jogging—2 minutes
- Push-Ups (Beginner or Intermediate)—1 minute (see pages 84–85)
- Jogging—2 minutes
- Hollywood One-Armed Row—1 minute (see page 93)
- Jogging—2 minutes
- Hollywood Bent-Over Rear Delt—1 minute (see page 103)
- Jogging—2 minutes
- Hollywood Ball Press—1 minute (see page 111)
- Jogging—2 minutes
- Pedal Your Waist Away—1 minute (see page 133)
- Rest—30 seconds
- Hollywood Crunch—1 minute (see page 129)
- Rest—30 seconds
- Hollywood Ball Crunch—1 minute (see page 135)
- Jogging—2 minutes

- Cleansing Minute (see pages 73–74)
- Jogging—2 minutes
- Intermediate Push-Up—1 minute (see page 85)
- Jogging—2 minutes
- Hollywood Ball Press—1 minute (see page 111)
- Jogging—2 minutes
- Hollywood Field Goals—1 minute (see page 101)
- Jogging—2 minutes
- Hollywood One-Armed Row—1 minute (see page 93)
- Jogging—2 minutes
- Hollywood Hammer Curl—1 minute (see page 107)
- Jogging—2 minutes
- Hollywood "I Dream of Jeannie" Squat—1 minute (see page 119)
- Jogging—2 minutes
- Hollywood Hamstring Curl—1 minute (see page 123)
- Jogging—2 minutes
- Hollywood Corkscrew—1 minute (see page 137)
- Rest—30 seconds
- Hollywood Crunch—1 minute (see page 129)
- Rest—30 seconds
- Side Plank with Hollywood Hip Raise—1 minute (see page 139)
- Jogging—2 minutes

Jogging Workout—Week Five, Workout Two

- Cleansing Minute (see pages 73–74)
- Jogging—2 minutes
- Hollywood Overhead Tri—1 minute (see page 113)
- Jogging—2 minutes
- Hollywood Bent-Over Rear Delt—1 minute (see page 103)
- Jogging—2 minutes
- Push-Ups (Beginner or Intermediate)—1 minute (see pages 84–85)
- Jogging—2 minutes
- Hollywood Pull-Over—1 minute (see page 95)
- Jogging—2 minutes
- Biceps Curl with a Hollywood Twist—1 minute (see page 106)
- Jogging—2 minutes
- Hollywood "I Dream of Jeannie" Squat—1 minute (see page 119)
- Jogging—2 minutes
- Hollywood Butt Kick—1 minute (see page 121)
- Jogging—2 minutes
- Hollywood Surfboard with Alternating Leg Lifts—1 minute (see page 138)
- Rest—30 seconds
- Side Plank with Hollywood Hip Raise—1 minute (see page 139)
- Rest—30 seconds
- Hollywood Leg Lift—1 minute (see page 136)
- Jogging—2 minutes

- Cleansing Minute (see pages 73–74)
- Jogging—2 minutes
- Hollywood Arrow—1 minute (see page 122)
- Jogging—2 minutes
- Hollywood Sumo Squat with Calf Raise—1 minute (see page 120)
- Jogging—2 minutes
- Hollywood Hamstring Curl—1 minute (see page 123)
- Jogging—2 minutes
- Hollywood Incline Fly—1 minute (see page 88)
- Jogging—2 minutes
- Hollywood One-Armed Row—1 minute (see page 93)
- Jogging—2 minutes
- Hollywood W Shoulders—1 minute (see page 100)
- Jogging—2 minutes
- Hollywood Kickback with a Twist—1 minute (see page 110)
- Jogging—2 minutes
- Pedal Your Waist Away—1 minute (see page 133)
- Rest—30 seconds
- Hollywood Surfboard with Alternating Leg Lifts—1 minute (see page 138)
- Rest—30 seconds
- Side Plank with Hollywood Hip Raise—1 minute (see page 139)
- Jogging—2 minutes

Jogging Workout—Week Five, Workout Three

- Cleansing Minute (see pages 73–74)
- Jogging—2 minutes
- Hollywood Arrow—1 minute (see page 122)
- Jogging—2 minutes
- Hollywood Squeeze Play—1 minute (see page 126)
- Jogging—2 minutes
- Hollywood Hamstring Curl—1 minute (see page 123)
- Jogging—2 minutes
- Hollywood Bent-Over Row—1 minute (see page 94)
- Jogging—2 minutes
- Hollywood Field Goals—1 minute (see page 101)
- Jogging—2 minutes
- Hollywood Kickback with a Twist—1 minute (see page 110)
- Jogging—2 minutes
- Hollywood Hammer Curl—1 minute (see page 107)
- Jogging—2 minutes
- Pedal Your Waist Away—1 minute (see page 133)
- Rest—30 seconds
- Hollywood Ball Small Sit-Up—1 minute (see page 132)
- Rest—30 seconds
- Hollywood Leg Lift—1 minute (see page 136)
- Jogging—2 minutes

- Cleansing Minute (see pages 73–74)
- Jogging—2 minutes
- Hollywood Overhead Tri—1 minute (see page 113)
- Jogging—2 minutes
- Hollywood Bent-Over Rear Delt—1 minute (see page 103)
- Jogging—2 minutes
- Hollywood Fly—1 minute (see page 87)
- Jogging—2 minutes
- Hollywood Bent-Over Row—1 minute (see page 94)
- Jogging—2 minutes
- Biceps Curl with a Hollywood Twist—1 minute (see page 106)
- Jogging—2 minutes
- Hollywood Arrow—1 minute (see page 122)
- Jogging—2 minutes
- Hollywood Sumo Squat with Calf Raise—1 minute (see page 120)
- Jogging—2 minutes
- Hollywood Ball Crunch—1 minute (see page 135)
- Rest—30 seconds
- Hollywood Leg Lift—1 minute (see page 136)
- Rest—30 seconds
- Hollywood Reaching Penguins—1 minute (see page 134)
- Jogging—2 minutes

Jogging Workout—Week Six, Workout One

Women

- Cleansing Minute (see pages 73–74)
- Jogging—2 minutes
- Hollywood Pull-Over—1 minute (see page 95)
- Jogging—2 minutes
- Hollywood Fly—1 minute (see page 87)
- Jogging—2 minutes
- Hollywood W Shoulders—1 minute (see page 100)
- Jogging—2 minutes
- Hollywood Ball Press—1 minute (see page 111)
- Jogging—2 minutes
- Biceps Curl with a Hollywood Twist—1 minute (see page 106)
- Jogging—2 minutes
- Hollywood Hamstring Curl—1 minute (see page 123)
- Jogging—2 minutes
- Hollywood Squeeze Play—1 minute (see page 126)
- Jogging—2 minutes
- Hollywood Corkscrew—1 minute (see page 137)
- Rest—30 seconds
- Hollywood Crunch—1 minute (see page 129)
- Rest—30 seconds
- Side Plank with Hollywood Hip Raise—1 minute (see page 139)
- Jogging—2 minutes

- Cleansing Minute (see pages 73–74)
- Jogging—2 minutes
- Hollywood Hamstring Curl—1 minute (see page 123)
- Jogging—2 minutes
- Hollywood Sumo Squat with Calf Raise—1 minute (see page 120)
- Jogging—2 minutes
- Hollywood Incline Fly—1 minute (see page 88)
- Jogging—2 minutes
- Hollywood Field Goals—1 minute (see page 101)
- Jogging—2 minutes
- Hollywood Pull-Over—1 minute (see page 93)
- Jogging—2 minutes
- Hollywood Ball Press—1 minute (see page 111)
- Jogging—2 minutes
- Hollywood Hammer Curl—1 minute (see page 107)
- Jogging—2 minutes
- Hollywood Ball Small Sit-Up—1 minute (see page 132)
- Rest—30 seconds
- Hollywood Surfboard with Alternating Leg Lifts—1 minute (see page 138)
- Rest—30 seconds
- Side Plank with Hollywood Hip Raise—1 minute (see page 139)
- Jogging—2 minutes

Jogging Workout—Week Six, Workout Two

- Cleansing Minute (see pages 73–74)
- Jogging—2 minutes
- Hollywood Sumo Squat with Calf Raise—1 minute (see page 120)
- Jogging—2 minutes
- Hollywood Side Raise—1 minute (see page 125)
- Jogging—2 minutes
- Hollywood Arrow—1 minute (see page 122)
- Jogging—2 minutes
- Hollywood Bent-Over Rear Delt—1 minute (see page 103)
- Jogging—2 minutes
- Hollywood One-Armed Row—1 minute (see page 93)
- Jogging—2 minutes
- Hollywood Overhead Tri—1 minute (see page 113)
- Jogging—2 minutes
- Push-Ups (Beginner or Intermediate)—1 minute (see pages 84–85)
- Jogging—2 minutes
- Hollywood Surfboard with Alternating Leg Lifts—1 minute (see page 138)
- Rest—30 seconds
- Hollywood Ball Crunch—1 minute (see page 135)
- Rest—30 seconds
- Hollywood Crossover Crunch—1 minute (see page 131)
- Jogging—2 minutes

- Cleansing Minute (see pages 73–74)
- Jogging—2 minutes
- Hollywood Pull-Over—1 minute (see page 95)
- Jogging—2 minutes
- Hollywood W Shoulders—1 minute (see page 100)
- Jogging—2 minutes
- Hollywood Overhead Tri—1 minute (see page 113)
- Jogging—2 minutes
- Biceps Curl with a Hollywood Twist—1 minute (see page 106)
- Jogging—2 minutes
- Hollywood Hamstring Curl—1 minute (see page 123)
- Jogging—2 minutes
- Hollywood Sumo Squat with Calf Raise—1 minute (see page 120)
- Jogging—2 minutes
- Hollywood Arrow—1 minute (see page 122)
- Jogging—2 minutes
- Hollywood Corkscrew—1 minute (see page 137)
- Rest—30 seconds
- Hollywood Crunch—1 minute (see page 129)
- Rest—30 seconds
- Hollywood Reaching Penguins—1 minute (see page 134)
- Jogging—2 minutes

Jogging Workout—Week Six, Workout Three

Women

- Cleansing Minute (see pages 73–74)
- Jogging—2 minutes
- Hollywood Hamstring Curl—1 minute (see page 123)
- Jogging—2 minutes
- Hollywood Arrow—1 minute (see page 122)
- Jogging—2 minutes
- Hollywood Squeeze Play—1 minute (see page 124)
- Jogging—2 minutes
- Hollywood Bent-Over Row—1 minute (see page 94)
- Jogging—2 minutes
- Hollywood Field Goals—1 minute (see page 101)
- Jogging—2 minutes
- Hollywood Kickback with a Twist—1 minute (see page 110)
- Jogging—2 minutes
- Hollywood Hammer Curl—1 minute (see page 107)
- Jogging—2 minutes
- Hollywood Crossover Crunch—1 minute (see page 131)
- Rest—30 seconds
- Hollywood Reaching Penguins—1 minute (see page 134)
- Rest—30 seconds
- Hollywood Leg Lift—1 minute (see page 136)
- Jogging—2 minutes

- Cleansing Minute (see pages 73–74)
- Jogging—2 minutes
- Hollywood Sumo Squat with Calf Raise—1 minute (see page 120)
- Jogging—2 minutes
- Hollywood Arrow—1 minute (see page 122)
- Jogging—2 minutes
- Intermediate Push-Up—1 minute (see page 85)
- Jogging—2 minutes
- Hollywood Ball Press—1 minute (see page 111)
- Jogging—2 minutes
- Hollywood Bent-Over Rear Delt—1 minute (see page 103)
- Jogging—2 minutes
- Hollywood Bent-Over Row—1 minute (see page 94)
- Jogging—2 minutes
- Hollywood Hammer Curl—1 minute (see page 107)
- Jogging—2 minutes
- Pedal Your Waist Away—1 minute (see page 133)
- Rest—30 seconds
- Hollywood Crunch—1 minute (see page 129)
- Rest—30 seconds
- Hollywood Ball Crunch—1 minute (see page 135)
- Jogging—2 minutes

Six-Week Measurements

Neck _____ Shoulders _____

Chest _____ Waist _____ Hips _____

Right biceps (flexed) _____ Left biceps (flexed) _____

Right thigh _____ Left thigh _____

Right calf _____ Left calf _____

Resting heart rate _____

Body fat percentage _____

10

The Celebrity Makeover Stepping Phase—Weeks 7 and 8

Y ou've done a super job! We're getting there! At this point, you should be able to see the light at the end of the tunnel.

Stepping

Our next phase will ramp things up even further. Now you're going to be stepping up and down on a platform. If you have a Reebok Step like the ones at the gym, that's great, but if you don't, don't worry—use the bottom step of a flight of stairs. Stepping will combine some of the dynamic movements of jogging with the higher leg lift and the greater range of motion of marching. And the sum is greater than the individual parts. In addition to getting the benefits of both jogging and marching—strengthening the hip flexors and calves and stretching the hip extensors—you'll also work on strengthening your glutes and your quadriceps in the front of your thighs. Remember that any time you take the leg from a bent-knee position to a straight-leg position, you're working your quads, and any time you take your body from a bent-at-the-hips position to a straight-body position, you're working your glutes. Every time you have to step up, you're

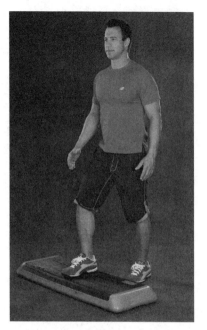

doing just that. Every step is a mini-one-legged squat. I want you to think how many times you'll be doing that over the course of each stepping workout. My guess is about a zillion. And all that stepping isn't only great for your thighs and butt; it also gets your heart rate up and burns calories like crazy.

Here's how I want you to do it: step up with the right foot, then up with the left, then down with the right, then down with the left. As far as the pace goes, I want you to go at a rate that will let you complete the entire 2 minutes without stopping. So, depending on your condition and how you feel on a particular day, the pace may be a fast or a slow one. Again, just do your best.

If you are using a Reebok Step or a similar piece of equipment, feel free to challenge yourself by adding risers that will elevate the step and force you to work a little harder. Initially, start with just the step and no risers. If you want, you can gradually work your way up to using three risers. Remember, I said gradually. Three risers will give you quite a workout.

I've done my best to get your legs ready for this phase of the program, so you should be good to go. If you do feel a little bit of soreness the day after a workout, though, that's pretty normal. As your body gets used to the motion, that soreness will lessen and eventually go away.

Checking In

For the first three phases, I threw in a few words of encouragement just before letting you head off to the workouts. I'm not going to do that this time because I know that if you've made it this far, you don't need it. The way you feel and the way you know you look should be motivation enough to keep you going. But if you think you look and feel great right now, just imagine what you'll feel like in another four weeks!

Stepping Workout—Week Seven, Workout One

- Cleansing Minute (see pages 73–74)
- Stepping—2 minutes
- Hollywood Arrow—1 minute (see page 122)
- Stepping—2 minutes
- Hollywood Zorro Lunge—1 minute (see page 124)
- Stepping—2 minutes
- Hollywood Side Raise—1 minute (see page 125)
- Stepping—2 minutes
- Hollywood One-Armed Row—1 minute (see page 93)
- Stepping—2 minutes
- Hollywood Field Goals—1 minute (see page 101)
- Stepping—2 minutes
- Hollywood Fly—1 minute (see page 87)
- Stepping—2 minutes
- Hollywood Ball Press—1 minute (see page 111)
- Stepping—2 minutes
- Hollywood Ball Small Sit-Up—1 minute (see page 132)
- Rest—30 seconds
- Hollywood Corkscrew—1 minute (see page 137)
- Rest—30 seconds
- Hollywood Ball Crunch—1 minute (see page 135)
- Stepping—2 minutes

- Cleansing Minute (see pages 73–74)
- Stepping—2 minutes
- Hollywood Zorro Lunge—1 minute (see page 124)
- Stepping—2 minutes
- Hollywood Hamstring Curl—1 minute (see page 123)
- Stepping—2 minutes
- Push-Ups (Intermediate or Advanced)—1 minute (see pages 85–86)
- Stepping—2 minutes
- Hollywood Shrug—1 minute (see page 96)
- Stepping—2 minutes
- Hollywood W Shoulders—1 minute (see page 100)
- Stepping—2 minutes
- Hollywood Overhead Tri—1 minute (see page 113)
- Stepping—2 minutes
- Hollywood Karate Curl—1 minute (see page 109)
- Stepping—2 minutes
- Pedal Your Waist Away—1 minute (see page 133)
- Rest—30 seconds
- Hollywood Crunch—1 minute (see page 129)
- Rest—30 seconds
- Hollywood Ball Crunch—1 minute (see page 135)
- Stepping—2 minutes

Stepping Workout—Week Seven, Workout Two

- Cleansing Minute (see pages 73–74)
- Stepping—2 minutes
- Hollywood Bent-Over Rear Delt—1 minute (see page 103)
- Stepping—2 minutes
- Hollywood Bent-Over Row—1 minute (see page 94)
- Stepping—2 minutes
- Hollywood Kickback with a Twist—1 minute (see page 110)
- Stepping—2 minutes
- Biceps Curl with a Hollywood Twist—1 minute (see page 106)
- Stepping—2 minutes
- Hollywood Squeeze Play—1 minute (see page 126)
- Stepping—2 minutes
- Hollywood Butt Kick—1 minute (see page 121)
- Stepping—2 minutes
- Hollywood Arrow—1 minute (see page 122)
- Stepping—2 minutes
- Hollywood Leg Lift—1 minute (see page 136)
- Rest—30 seconds
- Hollywood Surfboard with Alternating Leg Lifts—1 minute (see page 138)
- Rest—30 seconds
- Side Plank with Hollywood Hip Raise—1 minute (see page 139)
- Stepping—2 minutes

- Cleansing Minute (see pages 73–74)
- Stepping—2 minutes
- Hollywood Ball Press—1 minute (see page 111)
- Stepping—2 minutes
- Hollywood Bent-Over Rear Delt—1 minute (see page 103)
- Stepping—2 minutes
- Hollywood Incline Fly—1 minute (see page 88)
- Stepping—2 minutes
- Hollywood Karate Curl—1 minute (see page 109)
- Stepping—2 minutes
- Hollywood "I Dream of Jeannie" Squat—1 minute (see page 119)
- Stepping—2 minutes
- Hollywood Hamstring Curl—1 minute (see page 123)
- Stepping—2 minutes
- Hollywood Zorro Lunge—1 minute (see page 124)
- Stepping—2 minutes
- Hollywood Corkscrew—1 minute (see page 137)
- Rest—30 seconds
- Hollywood Surfboard with Alternating Leg Lifts—1 minute (see page 138)
- Rest—30 seconds
- Side Plank with Hollywood Hip Raise—1 minute (see page 139)
- Stepping—2 minutes

Stepping Workout—Week Seven, Workout Three

Women

- Cleansing Minute (see pages 73–74)
- Stepping—2 minutes
- Hollywood "I Dream of Jeannie" Squat—1 minute (see page 119)
- Stepping—2 minutes
- Hollywood Hamstring Curl—1 minute (see page 123)
- Stepping—2 minutes
- Hollywood Zorro Lunge—1 minute (see page 124)
- Stepping—2 minutes
- Hollywood W Shoulders—1 minute (see page 100)
- Stepping—2 minutes
- Intermediate Push-Up—1 minute (see page 85)
- Stepping—2 minutes
- Hollywood Overhead Tri—1 minute (see page 113)
- Stepping—2 minutes
- Hollywood Hammer Curl—1 minute (see page 107)
- Stepping—2 minutes
- Pedal Your Waist Away—1 minute (see page 133)
- Rest—30 seconds
- Hollywood Ball Small Sit-Up—1 minute (see page 132)
- Rest—30 seconds
- Hollywood Reaching Penguins—1 minute (see page 134)
- Stepping—2 minutes

- Cleansing Minute (see pages 73–74)
- Stepping—2 minutes
- Hollywood Fly—1 minute (see page 87)
- Stepping—2 minutes
- Hollywood Bent-Over Row—1 minute (see page 94)
- Stepping—2 minutes
- Hollywood Field Goals—1 minute (see page 101)
- Stepping—2 minutes
- Hollywood Hammer Curl—1 minute (see page 107)
- Stepping—2 minutes
- Hollywood Sumo Squat with Calf Raise—1 minute (see page 120)
- Stepping—2 minutes
- Hollywood Arrow—1 minute (see page 122)
- Stepping—2 minutes
- Hollywood Hamstring Curl—1 minute (see page 123)
- Stepping—2 minutes
- Hollywood Crossover Crunch—1 minute (see page 131)
- Rest—30 seconds
- Hollywood Reaching Penguins—1 minute (see page 134)
- Rest—30 seconds
- Hollywood Leg Lift—1 minute (see page 137)
- Stepping—2 minutes

Stepping Workout—Week Eight, Workout One

Women

- Cleansing Minute (see pages 73–74)
- Stepping—2 minutes
- Hollywood Field Goals—1 minute (see page 101)
- Stepping—2 minutes
- Hollywood Kickback with a Twist—1 minute (see page 110)
- Stepping—2 minutes
- Hollywood Fly—1 minute (see page 87)
- Stepping—2 minutes
- Hollywood Pull-Over—1 minute (see page 95)
- Stepping—2 minutes
- Hollywood Zorro Lunge—1 minute (see page 124)
- Stepping—2 minutes
- Hollywood Hamstring Curl—1 minute (see page 123)
- Stepping—2 minutes
- Hollywood Arrow—1 minute (see page 122)
- Stepping—2 minutes
- Hollywood Ball Crunch—1 minute (see page 135)
- Rest—30 seconds
- Hollywood Crunch—1 minute (see page 129)
- Rest—30 seconds
- Side Plank with Hollywood Hip Raise—1 minute (see page 139)
- Stepping—2 minutes

- Cleansing Minute (see pages 73–74)
- Stepping—2 minutes
- Hollywood Arrow—1 minute (see page 122)
- Stepping—2 minutes
- Hollywood Zorro Lunge—1 minute (see page 124)
- Stepping—2 minutes
- Hollywood Sumo Squat with Calf Raise—1 minute (see page 120)
- Stepping—2 minutes
- Push-Ups (Intermediate or Advanced)—1 minute (see pages 85–86)
- Stepping—2 minutes
- Hollywood Ball Press—1 minute (see page 111)
- Stepping—2 minutes
- Hollywood W Shoulders—1 minute (see page 100)
- Stepping—2 minutes
- Hollywood Hammer Curl—1 minute (see page 107)
- Stepping—2 minutes
- Hollywood Ball Crunch—1 minute (see page 135)
- Rest—30 seconds
- Pedal Your Waist Away—1 minute (see page 133)
- Rest—30 seconds
- Hollywood Leg Lift—1 minute (see page 136)
- Stepping—2 minutes

Stepping Workout—Week Eight, Workout Two

- Cleansing Minute (see pages 73–74)
- Stepping—2 minutes
- Hollywood Squeeze Play—1 minute (see page 126)
- Stepping—2 minutes
- Hollywood Sumo Squat with Calf Raise—1 minute (see page 120)
- Stepping—2 minutes
- Hollywood Arrow—1 minute (see page 122)
- Stepping—2 minutes
- Hollywood Shrug—1 minute (see page 96)
- Stepping—2 minutes
- Intermediate Push-Up—1 minute (see page 85)
- Stepping—2 minutes
- Hollywood Bent-Over Rear Delt—1 minute (see page 103)
- Stepping—2 minutes
- Hollywood Overhead Tri—1 minute (see page 113)
- Stepping—2 minutes
- Hollywood Crossover Crunch—1 minute (see page 131)
- Rest—30 seconds
- Hollywood Surfboard with Alternating Leg Lifts—1 minute (see page 136)
- Rest—30 seconds
- Hollywood Leg Lift—1 minute (see page 136)
- Stepping—2 minutes

- Cleansing Minute (see pages 73–74)
- Stepping—2 minutes
- Hollywood Field Goals—1 minute (see page 101)
- Stepping—2 minutes
- Hollywood Incline Fly—1 minute (see page 88)
- Stepping—2 minutes
- Hollywood Bent-Over Row—1 minute (see page 94)
- Stepping—2 minutes
- Hollywood Kickback with a Twist—1 minute (see page 110)
- Stepping—2 minutes
- Hollywood Karate Curl—1 minute (see page 109)
- Stepping—2 minutes
- Hollywood Hamstring Curl—1 minute (see page 123)
- Stepping—2 minutes
- Hollywood "I Dream of Jeannie" Squat—1 minute (see page 119)
- Stepping—2 minutes
- One-Legged Hollywood Crunch—1 minute (see page 130)
- Rest—30 seconds
- Hollywood Surfboard with Alternating Leg Lifts—1 minute (see page 138)
- Rest—30 seconds
- Side Plank with Hollywood Hip Raise—1 minute (see page 139)
- Stepping—2 minutes

Stepping Workout—Week Eight, Workout Three

- Cleansing Minute (see pages 73–74)
- Stepping—2 minutes
- Hollywood One-Armed Row—1 minute (see page 93)
- Stepping—2 minutes
- Hollywood W Shoulders—1 minute (see page 100)
- Stepping—2 minutes
- Hollywood Incline Fly—1 minute (see page 88)
- Stepping—2 minutes
- Hollywood Ball Press—1 minute (see page 111)
- Stepping—2 minutes
- Hollywood Sumo Squat with Calf Raise—1 minute (see page 120)
- Stepping—2 minutes
- Hollywood Hamstring Curl—1 minute (see page 123)
- Stepping—2 minutes
- Hollywood Squeeze Play—1 minute (see page 126)
- Stepping—2 minutes
- Side Plank with Hollywood Hip Raise—1 minute (see page 139)
- Rest—30 seconds
- Hollywood Corkscrew—1 minute (see page 137)
- Rest—30 seconds
- Hollywood Crunch—1 minute (see page 129)
- Stepping—2 minutes

- Cleansing Minute (see pages 73–74)
- Stepping—2 minutes
- Hollywood Zorro Lunge—1 minute (see page 124)
- Stepping—2 minutes
- Hollywood Hamstring Curl—1 minute (see page 123)
- Stepping—2 minutes
- Hollywood Pull-Over—1 minute (see page 95)
- Stepping—2 minutes
- Hollywood W Shoulders—1 minute (see page 100)
- Stepping—2 minutes
- Hollywood Overhead Tri—1 minute (see page 113)
- Stepping—2 minutes
- Hollywood Incline Fly—1 minute (see page 88)
- Stepping—2 minutes
- Biceps Curl with a Hollywood Twist—1 minute (see page 106)
- Stepping—2 minutes
- Hollywood Ball Small Sit-Up—1 minute (see page 132)
- Rest—30 seconds
- Hollywood Corkscrew—1 minute (see page 137)
- Rest—30 seconds
- Hollywood Ball Crunch—1 minute (see page 133)
- Stepping—2 minutes

Eight-Week Measurements

Neck _____ Shoulders _____

Chest _____ Waist _____ Hips _____

Right biceps (flexed) _____ Left biceps (flexed) _____

Right thigh _____ Left thigh _____

Right calf _____ Left calf _____

Resting heart rate _____

Body fat percentage _____

11

The Celebrity Makeover Lunging Phase— Weeks 9 and 10

You're in the home stretch! By now, you should be looking and feeling great, and you have only two weeks to go.

I'm not going to let you coast to the finish line, though. You'll have to earn it. The last phase is the most challenging. You've walked, marched, jogged, stepped, and now you're going to lunge.

Lunging

Lunging is just about the best body-weight exercise you can do. It works pretty much everything in your lower body and your core while improving your balance and body awareness. Not bad, huh?

Before I tell you just how good lunges are for you, let me tell you how I want you to do them. The key to lunging is good form. It'll make sure you target the muscles you want and avoid the chance of injury. Here's the deal.

Start with your feet hip-width apart and with your hands on your hips. Inhale and slowly step out deeply with your right foot. In this lunging position, it's very important that your right knee is centered

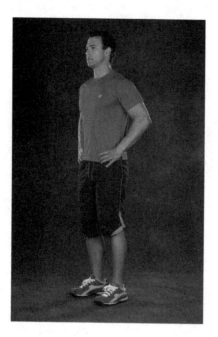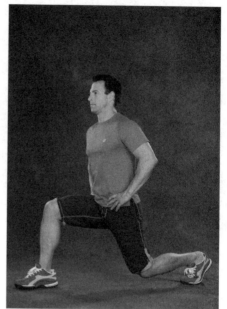

over your right heel and that your left knee doesn't touch the ground. Try not to lean forward. Maintaining good posture is a good way to keep your knees where they should be. Push off the right foot as you exhale to return to the starting position. Now lunge with the left leg.

Every time you step forward into the lunge position, you're giving a great stretch to the hip flexor of the trailing leg. You're also working the hamstrings of the lead leg because it's their job to stabilize the body and keep you from falling forward. When you push back up to the starting position, you're doing a dynamic one-legged leg press, which you'll feel in your quads and glutes. Meanwhile, the entire time you're forced to keep your abs and lower back engaged so that you don't fall over. This strengthens your core while improving your overall sense of balance.

Again, form is the key when it comes to doing lunges. If at any time you find your form slipping, switch to either jogging or stepping.

Strength Training

In this last phase of the program I pull out all the stops. You've gone from doing some very basic strength training movements to doing some very complex ones. Just as with the cardio portion of the program, we started with the basics. Again, you literally walked before you could run. If there were some strength-training motions that you originally found too challenging, my hope is that you've gone back to try them and have found them a lot more doable. There may even be some exercises that you originally hated to do—we all have those—but that you now can't wait to do. This is tangible evidence of how positively your body has responded to the workouts. You've gotten stronger, more fit, and, maybe most important, better able to use your own body. This is in addition to losing weight, feeling great, and looking, quite possibly, the best you ever have.

That brand-new Hollywood you is just two weeks away!

Lunging Workout—Week Nine, Workout One

- Cleansing Minute (see pages 73–74)
- Lunging—2 minutes
- Hollywood Hamstring Curl—1 minute (see page 123)
- Lunging—2 minutes
- Hollywood Squeeze Play—1 minute (see page 126)
- Lunging—2 minutes
- Advanced Push-Up—1 minute (see page 86)
- Lunging—2 minutes
- Hollywood Pull-Over—1 minute (see page 95)
- Lunging—2 minutes
- Hollywood Funky Chicken—1 minute (see page 102)
- Lunging—2 minutes
- Hollywood Ball Press—1 minute (see page 111)
- Lunging—2 minutes
- Hollywood Upside-Down Curl—1 minute (see page 108)
- Lunging—2 minutes
- Hollywood Ball Crunch—1 minute (see page 135)
- Rest—30 seconds
- Hollywood Corkscrew—1 minute (see page 137)
- Rest—30 seconds
- Hollywood Ball Small Sit-Up—1 minute (see page 132)
- Lunging—2 minutes

- Cleansing Minute (see pages 73–74)
- Lunging—2 minutes
- Hollywood C Sweep—1 minute (see page 89)
- Lunging—2 minutes
- Hollywood Hyperextension—1 minute (see page 97)
- Lunging—2 minutes
- Hollywood Field Goals—1 minute (see page 101)
- Lunging—2 minutes
- Alternating Hollywood Triceps Raise—1 minute (see page 112)
- Lunging—2 minutes
- Hollywood Upside-Down Curl—1 minute (see page 108)
- Lunging—2 minutes
- Hollywood Arrow—1 minute (see page 122)
- Lunging—2 minutes
- Hollywood "I Dream of Jeannie" Squat—1 minute (see page 119)
- Lunging—2 minutes
- Hollywood Ball Small Sit-Up—1 minute (see page 132)
- Rest—30 seconds
- Hollywood Reaching Penguins—1 minute (see page 134)
- Rest—30 seconds
- Hollywood Leg Lift—1 minute (see page 136)
- Lunging—2 minutes

Lunging Workout—Week Nine, Workout Two

- Cleansing Minute (see pages 73–74)
- Lunging—2 minutes
- Hollywood Hamstring Curl—1 minute (see page 123)
- Lunging—2 minutes
- Hollywood Arrow—1 minute (see page 122)
- Lunging—2 minutes
- Hollywood C Sweep—1 minute (see page 89)
- Lunging—2 minutes
- Hollywood Hyperextension—1 minute (see page 97)
- Lunging—2 minutes
- Hollywood Field Goals—1 minute (see page 101)
- Lunging—2 minutes
- Hollywood Overhead Tri—1 minute (see page 113)
- Lunging—2 minutes
- Biceps Curl with a Hollywood Twist—1 minute (see page 106)
- Lunging—2 minutes
- Hollywood Surfboard with Alternating Leg Lifts—1 minute (see page 138)
- Rest—30 seconds
- Side Plank with Hollywood Hip Raise—1 minute (see page 139)
- Rest—30 seconds
- Hollywood Crossover Crunch—1 minute (see page 131)
- Lunging—2 minutes

- Cleansing Minute (see pages 73–74)
- Lunging—2 minutes
- Hollywood Arrow—1 minute (see page 122)
- Lunging—2 minutes
- Hollywood Hamstring Curl—1 minute (see page 123)
- Lunging—2 minutes
- Advanced Push-Up—1 minute (see page 86)
- Lunging—2 minutes
- Hollywood Field Goals—1 minute (see page 101)
- Lunging—2 minutes
- Hollywood Kickback with a Twist—1 minute (see page 110)
- Lunging—2 minutes
- Hollywood Shrug—1 minute (see page 96)
- Lunging—2 minutes
- Hollywood Karate Curl—1 minute (see page 109)
- Lunging—2 minutes
- Hollywood Corkscrew—1 minute (see page 137)
- Rest—30 seconds
- Hollywood Ball Small Sit-Up—1 minute (see page 132)
- Rest—30 seconds
- Hollywood Surfboard with Alternating Leg Lifts—1 minute (see page 138)
- Lunging—2 minutes

Lunging Workout—Week Nine, Workout Three

Women

- Cleansing Minute (see pages 73–74)
- Lunging—2 minutes
- Advanced Push-Up—1 minute (see page 86)
- Lunging—2 minutes
- Hollywood Overhead Tri—1 minute (see page 113)
- Lunging—2 minutes
- Hollywood One-Armed Row—1 minute (see page 93)
- Lunging—2 minutes
- Hollywood Funky Chicken—1 minute (see page 102)
- Lunging—2 minutes
- Hollywood Upside-Down Curl—1 minute (see page 108)
- Lunging—2 minutes
- Hollywood Butt Kick—1 minute (see page 121)
- Lunging—2 minutes
- Hollywood Arrow—1 minute (see page 122)
- Lunging—2 minutes
- Hollywood Leg Lift—1 minute (see page 136)
- Rest—30 seconds
- Pedal Your Waist Away—1 minute (see page 133)
- Rest—30 seconds
- Hollywood Ball Crunch—1 minute (see page 135)
- Lunging—2 minutes

- Cleansing Minute (see pages 73–74)
- Lunging—2 minutes
- Hollywood C Sweep—1 minute (see page 89)
- Lunging—2 minutes
- Hollywood Bent-Over Row—1 minute (see page 94)
- Lunging—2 minutes
- Hollywood Funky Chicken—1 minute (see page 102)
- Lunging—2 minutes
- Hollywood Ball Press—1 minute (see page 111)
- Lunging—2 minutes
- Hollywood Hammer Curl—1 minute (see page 107)
- Lunging—2 minutes
- Hollywood Sumo Squat with Calf Raise—1 minute (see page 120)
- Lunging—2 minutes
- Hollywood Hamstring Curl—1 minute (see page 123)
- Lunging—2 minutes
- Pedal Your Waist Away—1 minute (see page 133)
- Rest—30 seconds
- Hollywood Corkscrew—1 minute (see page 137)
- Rest—30 seconds
- Hollywood Reaching Penguins—1 minute (see page 134)
- Lunging—2 minutes

Lunging Workout—Week Ten, Workout One

Women

- Cleansing Minute (see pages 73–74)
- Lunging—2 minutes
- Hollywood Hamstring Curl—1 minute (see page 123)
- Lunging—2 minutes
- Hollywood Squeeze Play—1 minute (see page 126)
- Lunging—2 minutes
- Hollywood Hyperextension—1 minute (see page 97)
- Lunging—2 minutes
- Hollywood Bent-Over Rear Delt—1 minute (see page 103)
- Lunging—2 minutes
- Hollywood Shrug—1 minute (see page 96)
- Lunging—2 minutes
- Hollywood Kickback with a Twist—1 minute (see page 110)
- Lunging—2 minutes
- Biceps Curl with a Hollywood Twist—1 minute (see page 106)
- Lunging—2 minutes
- Hollywood Reaching Penguins—1 minute (see page 134)
- Rest—30 seconds
- Hollywood Ball Small Sit-Up—1 minute (see page 132)
- Rest—30 seconds
- Side Plank with Hollywood Hip Raise—1 minute (see page 139)
- Lunging—2 minutes

- Cleansing Minute (see pages 73–74)
- Lunging—2 minutes
- Hollywood Sumo Squat with Calf Raise—1 minute (see page 120)
- Lunging—2 minutes
- Hollywood Arrow—1 minute (see page 122)
- Lunging—2 minutes
- Advanced Push-Up—1 minute (see page 86)
- Lunging—2 minutes
- Hollywood Shrug—1 minute (see page 96)
- Lunging—2 minutes
- Hollywood W Shoulders—1 minute (see page 100)
- Lunging—2 minutes
- Hollywood Overhead Tri—1 minute (see page 113)
- Lunging—2 minutes
- Hollywood Karate Curl—1 minute (see page 109)
- Lunging—2 minutes
- Pedal Your Waist Away—1 minute (see page 133)
- Rest—30 seconds
- One-Legged Hollywood Crunch—1 minute (see page 130)
- Rest—30 seconds
- Side Plank with Hollywood Hip Raise—1 minute (see page 139)
- Lunging—2 minutes

Lunging Workout—Week Ten, Workout Two

- Cleansing Minute (see pages 73–74)
- Lunging—2 minutes
- Hollywood Pull-Over—1 minute (see page 95)
- Lunging—2 minutes
- Hollywood Fly—1 minute (see page 87)
- Lunging—2 minutes
- Hollywood Field Goals—1 minute (see page 101)
- Lunging—2 minutes
- Alternating Hollywood Triceps Raise—1 minute (see page 112)
- Lunging—2 minutes
- Hollywood Hammer Curl—1 minute (see page 107)
- Lunging—2 minutes
- Hollywood Butt Kick—1 minute (see page 121)
- Lunging—2 minutes
- Hollywood Squeeze Play—1 minute (see page 126)
- Lunging—2 minutes
- Hollywood Ball Crunch—1 minute (see page 135)
- Rest—30 seconds
- Hollywood Corkscrew—1 minute (see page 137)
- Rest—30 seconds
- Hollywood Ball Small Sit-Up—1 minute (see page 132)
- Lunging—2 minutes

- Cleansing Minute (see pages 73–74)
- Lunging—2 minutes
- Hollywood Pull-Over—1 minute (see page 95)
- Lunging—2 minutes
- Hollywood W Shoulders—1 minute (see page 100)
- Lunging—2 minutes
- Hollywood Ball Press—1 minute (see page 111)
- Lunging—2 minutes
- Hollywood Incline Fly—1 minute (see page 88)
- Lunging—2 minutes
- Biceps Curl with a Hollywood Twist—1 minute (see page 106)
- Lunging—2 minutes
- Hollywood "I Dream of Jeannie" Squat—1 minute (see page 119)
- Lunging—2 minutes
- Hollywood Hamstring Curl—1 minute (see page 123)
- Lunging—2 minutes
- Hollywood Ball Crunch—1 minute (see page 135)
- Rest—30 seconds
- Hollywood Corkscrew—1 minute (see page 137)
- Rest—30 seconds
- Hollywood Ball Small Sit-Up—1 minute (see page 132)
- Lunging—2 minutes

Lunging Workout—Week Ten, Workout Three

Women

- Cleansing Minute (see pages 73–74)
- Lunging—2 minutes
- Hollywood Hamstring Curl—1 minute (see page 123)
- Lunging—2 minutes
- Hollywood "I Dream of Jeannie" Squat—1 minute (see page 119)
- Lunging—2 minutes
- Hollywood Ball Press—1 minute (see page 111)
- Lunging—2 minutes
- Hollywood Fly—1 minute (see page 87)
- Lunging—2 minutes
- Hollywood Bent-Over Row—1 minute (see page 94)
- Lunging—2 minutes
- Hollywood Funky Chicken—1 minute (see page 102)
- Lunging—2 minutes
- Hollywood Upside-Down Curl—1 minute (see page 108)
- Lunging—2 minutes
- Side Plank with Hollywood Hip Raise—1 minute (see page 139)
- Rest—30 seconds
- Pedal Your Waist Away—1 minute (see page 133)
- Rest—30 seconds
- Hollywood Surfboard with Alternating Leg Lifts—1 minute (see page 138)
- Lunging—2 minutes

- Cleansing Minute (see pages 73–74)
- Lunging—2 minutes
- Hollywood Arrow—1 minute (see page 122)
- Lunging—2 minutes
- Hollywood Sumo Squat with Calf Raise—1 minute (see page 120)
- Lunging—2 minutes
- Hollywood One-Armed Row—1 minute (see page 93)
- Lunging—2 minutes
- Hollywood C Sweep—1 minute (see page 89)
- Lunging—2 minutes
- Hollywood Funky Chicken—1 minute (see page 102)
- Lunging—2 minutes
- Alternating Hollywood Triceps Raise—1 minute (see page 113)
- Lunging—2 minutes
- Hollywood Upside-Down Curl—1 minute (see page 108)
- Lunging—2 minutes
- Hollywood Leg Lift—1 minute (see page 136)
- Rest—30 seconds
- Hollywood Surfboard with Alternating Leg Lifts—1 minute (see page 138)
- Rest—30 seconds
- Pedal Your Waist Away—1 minute (see page 133)
- Lunging—2 minutes

Final Measurements

Neck _____ Shoulders _____

Chest _____ Waist _____ Hips _____

Right biceps (flexed) _____ Left biceps (flexed) _____

Right thigh _____ Left thigh _____

Right calf _____ Left calf _____

Resting heart rate _____

Body fat percentage _____

12

The Celebrity Makeover RAW Workout

I do a lot of business traveling. I'm constantly shuttling between L.A., where I have my home and gym, and New York, where I do my *Weekend Today* show pieces. And when I have a book to promote, I can be all over the place. I enjoy working out when I'm on the road. It helps me to stay focused on what I have to do and ensures that I stay in the best shape I can be in. The trouble is that when you check into a hotel, you're usually at the mercy of the fitness equipment they have—and a lot of the time, it's not so great.

That's why I came up with the Celebrity Makeover RAW Workout. It stands for Resistance and Walking. The idea, not unlike the idea behind the 30-Minute Celebrity Makeover Miracle, is that if I can combine my cardio and my strength training, I can cut down on the time I have to be in the gym. I can still get a solid workout but in a fraction of the time. On most of my business trips, I don't have the luxury of being able to spend all day in the gym.

Turn Your Treadmill into a Gym

The Celebrity Makeover RAW Workout uses resistance bands that attach to the handles of most treadmills and stationary bikes. I designed them myself. Using these bands, you're able to do a complete upper-body workout while you work your legs on the treadmill. Just like with the 30-Minute Celebrity Makeover Miracle, you no longer have to decide whether it's going to be cardio or strength training if you have only a half-hour to exercise.

It's not only the business traveler who can take advantage of my RAW Bands. I've given them to clients who do a lot of business travel—clients whom I didn't want to miss a workout just because they were on the road—and an interesting thing happened. They began using them during their regular cardio routines when they got back, and they started to get results that surprised even me.

The secret is that the body is constantly moving while you work out. These are small motions that are done with light resistance but are done continuously. The result is not bulky muscle but lean, strong muscle.

The only thing you need is a treadmill or a stationary bike that has a solid bar for a handle. (Open handles may lead to the bands slipping off.)

Check out some of the RAW workout exercises on the next few pages. And if you want to order a pair of bands or just want some more information about them, go to my Web site, atighteru.com.

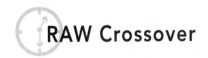

RAW Crossover

MUSCLE GROUP WORKED
This works the chest muscles.

GET READY
With a handle in each hand, have your forearms parallel to the floor at just-below chest level and your elbows extended slightly in front of your body.

DO THE EXERCISE
Take a deep breath. Exhale and slowly cross your right wrist over your left wrist in front of you as you squeeze your chest muscles together. Take a full three-count to do this. Hold for a beat, then take a three-count to return to the starting position as you inhale. Repeat, this time crossing your left wrist over the right. Do 20 reps at this pace.

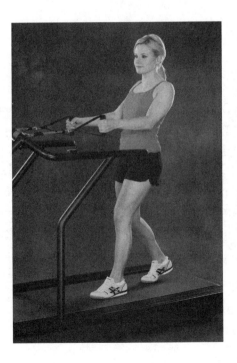
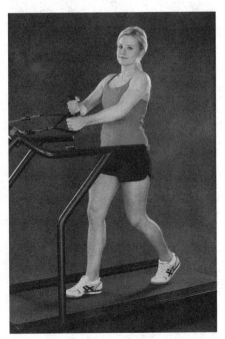

RAW Row

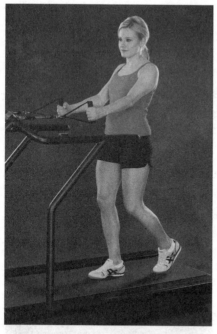

MUSCLE GROUP WORKED

This works the back muscles.

GET READY

Step back on the treadmill slightly so that you can extend your arms in front of you and still feel some tension in the RAW Bands. Your arms should be extended at just-below chest level with your palms facing each other.

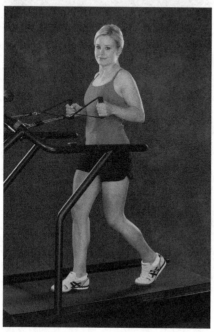

DO THE EXERCISE

Take a deep breath. Exhale and slowly draw the handles back away from the front of the treadmill by squeezing your shoulder blades together and drawing your elbows back. It should be a very smooth motion, not a jerking one. Take a three-count to do this. Hold for a beat, and return to the starting position over a three-count as you inhale.

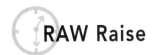

RAW Raise

MUSCLE GROUP WORKED

This works the shoulders muscles.

GET READY

Position yourself so that your upper arms are by your sides and your elbows are bent at 90-degree angles with your forearms extended toward the front of the treadmill and parallel to the floor. Your palms should be facing each other.

DO THE EXERCISE

Take a deep breath. Exhale and slowly, using a three-count, raise your elbows up to the sides. When your upper arms are parallel to the floor and your palms are facing the floor, hold for a beat and then slowly, over a three-count, lower your arms back to the starting position.

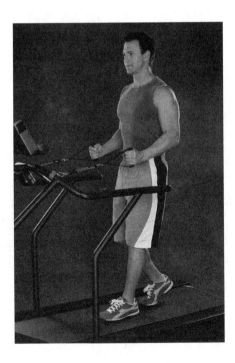
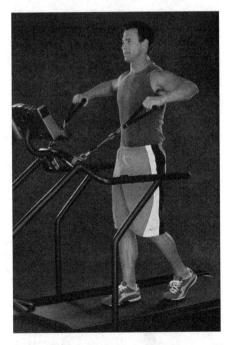

RAW Curl

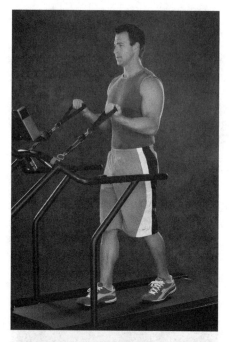

MUSCLE GROUP WORKED
This exercise works the biceps.

GET READY
Position yourself so that your upper arms are by your sides and your elbows are bent at 90-degree angles, with your forearms extended toward the front of the treadmill and parallel to the floor. Your palms should be facing up, and you should feel a fair amount of resistance from the bands.

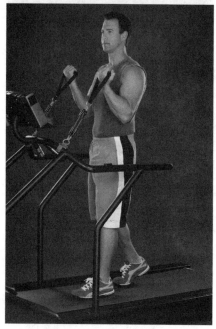

DO THE EXERCISE
Take a deep breath. Exhale and slowly raise the handles toward your shoulders by bending at the elbows. Keep your upper arms against your sides and try not to let them move. Go slowly, using a three-count. At the top of the motion, hold for a beat and reverse the movement over a three-count to return to the starting position as you inhale.

RAW Pressdown

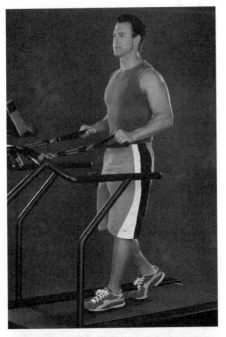

MUSCLE GROUP WORKED

This exercise works the triceps.

GET READY

Have your upper arms by your sides but flared out slightly. Your elbows should be bent at 90-degree angles so that your forearms are extended toward the front of the treadmill and are parallel to the floor. Your palms should be facing down.

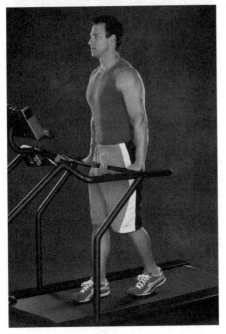

DO THE EXERCISE

Take a deep breath. Exhale and slowly press the handles down by your sides, straightening your arms. Take a full three-count to do this and avoid moving your upper arms. Lock your elbows at the bottom of the movement, hold for a beat, then return to the starting position over a three-count as you inhale.

13

Your New Present and Future

Guess what? You did it. You've transformed your body and your life. You're leaner, stronger, and more fit. Congratulations on sticking with the program, and thank you for letting me help you make some seriously positive changes.

I'll bet you've learned some things about yourself along the way. Sure, you now know the proper form for a biceps curl, but you've probably learned more than that. I'll bet you found out that you were tougher than you thought. I'll bet you discovered that you had more discipline than you thought. I'll bet you realized that you had more willpower than you thought. I would have told you in the first chapter that if you stuck with me, you'd learn all this, but I didn't want you to think I was being melodramatic.

The human spirit is an amazing thing. It's not always the stuff of epic movies. You don't have to save the kingdom from a gang of marauders or single-handedly overcome some ultimate evil. The human spirit can be exhibited simply by making it through an awful day at work, and instead of giving in to the temptation of eating a pint of ice cream, you take a few deep breaths and do your marching workout. It can be dealing with an upsetting phone call from an annoying relative, and instead of calling up anyone who'll listen to you vent, you focus yourself and do your lunging workout. By prioritizing things in your life and persevering when things might not have been so great, you've done more than just change the way you look; you've learned how to better handle your emotions and responsibilities. You've built more than just your body; you've built character.

Now What?

It's up to you. Right now, you're in good-enough shape to do just about anything. Getting fit is an incredibly liberating thing. If you've always wanted to do a walking tour of Italy but felt that you didn't have the stamina, guess what? You do now. If you've always wanted to take up tennis but didn't know whether your body was up to it, guess what? It is now. If you've always wanted to train for a 2K or 5K race but didn't know whether your muscles and joints could handle it, guess what? They can now.

I want you to go out and enjoy the fruits of your hard work. Go out and have fun with your new body. I want you to stay active. Do you realize how good you feel right now? Do you ever not want to feel this way?

If you want to continue working out with my program, feel free. You'll only feel better and better as time goes on. Continuing with my program is easy. You can go back and start with the first workout you did and progress from there, with one difference. No more walking or marching for you. You're beyond that, fitness-wise. No pun intended, but walking or marching, at this point, would be a step in the wrong direction. Start with the strength-training exercises that are part of the walking workout, but substitute jogging for walking. Do this for two weeks, then switch to stepping and then lunging. Your body will continue to be challenged and will continue to change.

A New You—a New Lifestyle

What I hope I've done is given you more than just a new body. I hope I've given you a love for fitness and for living a healthier life. I want you to love the feeling you get when you've just finished a tough workout. I want you to love the prospect of an even tougher workout two days later. I want you to love that feeling of accomplishment you get when you've done something that you never imagined you'd be able to do.

I've never spent a single dollar on advertising my studio; I've never had to. Why buy an ad in the newspaper or come up with a corny TV or radio ad when every one of my clients is a walking, breathing, living, three-dimensional, completely interactive advertisement for the benefits of a fit lifestyle? And guess what? Now you are, too.

We are living in one of the wealthiest nations in the world, yet most of us are woefully unfit. I need you to go out and spread the word. Not about me or my program, but about fitness. We need more people to be ambassadors of fitness. Your friends, family, and coworkers have already seen what a healthy lifestyle has done for you. And I guarantee that they've seen more than merely the physical benefits. They've seen you become more confident, more positive, and more grounded as well. If they're on the fence about getting started on a healthier lifestyle, I need you to gently knock them off that fence. And with all the strength training you've been doing, this should be easy.

Early on, I told you that this was a partnership—that I would give you everything you needed to change your life and what I needed in return was a promise of your commitment. Well, I need something else. I need you to go out once a week and go for a walk with someone who otherwise would have sat at his or her desk or on the couch. Your road to a new you began with walking, and I want you to show someone else that his or hers can, too. If we all try to reach out to as many people as we can, we can make the world a whole lot healthier.

I don't want to keep you. You didn't spend the last ten weeks working out just to hear me rambling. I'm sure there are things you want to do with your new body that are a lot more fun than reading a book.

Now go out and do them!

Resources

If you're having trouble finding any of the equipment or apparel you need, here are a few online sources:

www.power-systems.com
www.fitnessfactory.com
www.fitness1st.com
www.newbalance.com
www.adidas.com
www.nike.com

If you're looking for more information about Steve Zim, his studio, or his RAW bands, go to www.atighteru.com. If you're looking for more information about Steve Steinberg and his studio, check out www.blackbeltfitness.com. If you would like more information about the photography of Nicolas Sage, visit www.nicolassage.com.

Index